Principles of Basic Trauma Nursing

2nd Edition

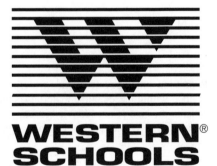

WESTERN® SCHOOLS

By
Brita M. O'Carroll, RN, BS, MEd, CPUR
Revised By
Judy Mikhail, RN, MSN, MBA

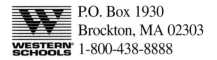

P.O. Box 1930
Brockton, MA 02303
1-800-438-8888

ABOUT THE ORIGINATING AUTHOR

Brita M. O'Carroll, RN, BS, MEd, CPUR, was educated at Duke University, Columbia University, New York University, and the University of North Florida. She has experience in clinical nursing, health information management, as an educator, a regional director for emergency medical services, international research, and is a published freelance writer. Ms. O'Carroll has made presentations at national and international conferences and is a Fellow in the Royal Society for the Promotion of Health and the International Council on Alcohol and Addictions.

ABOUT THE REVISING AUTHOR

Judy Mikhail, RN, MSN, MBA is Administrator for Trauma Services, Operating Room and Anesthesia at Hurley Medical Center, Flint, Michigan. She has 10 years of experience as Trauma Program Manager for a Level I Trauma Center as well as another 10 years of experience as a Clinical Nurse Specialist for trauma and critical care. Ms. Mikhail is an adjunct instructor at the University of Michigan-Flint School of Nursing, BSN Program. She has served as President of the Society of Trauma Nurses and The Michigan Trauma Coalition. She was selected by two consecutive Michigan Governors to serve on the Michigan Trauma Commission and the Michigan Trauma EMS Subcommittee. Ms. Mikhail has published numerous articles and speaks nationally on trauma related topics.

Judy Mikhail has disclosed that she has no significant financial or other conflicts of interest pertaining to this course book.

ABOUT THE SUBJECT MATTER REVIEWER

Patricia A. Manion, RN, MS, CCRN, CEN, is an experienced educator, critical care nurse, and trauma nurse. Her clinical and educator experience have included over 25 years of critical care in surgical, medical, and cardiac critical care units. Currently she is a Trauma Program Manager, a position she has held for over 9 years in two American College of Surgeons verified Trauma Centers. She is also currently the President of the Michigan State Council of the Emergency Nurses Association and a Trauma Nurse Certification Course Instructor and State Faculty. She received the Emergency Nurse Excellence Award for 2004 from the Michigan Emergency Nurses Association (ENA). She is also an active member of the Society of Trauma Nurses. Ms. Manion has taught hundreds of new trauma nurses throughout the state of Michigan and has presented trauma lectures in Michigan and at the National ENA Scientific Assembly.

Patricia A. Manion has disclosed that she has no significant financial or other conflicts of interest pertaining to this course book.

Nurse Planner: Amy Bernard, RN, BSN, MS

Copy Editor: Julie Munden

Indexer: Sylvia Coates

Western Schools' courses are designed to provide nursing professionals with the educational information they need to enhance their career development. The information provided within these course materials is the result of research and consultation with prominent nursing and medical authorities and is, to the best of our knowledge, current and accurate. However, the courses and course materials are provided with the understanding that Western Schools is not engaged in offering legal, nursing, medical, or other professional advice.

Western Schools' courses and course materials are not meant to act as a substitute for seeking out professional advice or conducting individual research. When the information provided in the courses and course materials is applied to individual circumstances, all recommendations must be considered in light of the uniqueness pertaining to each situation.

Western Schools' course materials are intended solely for *your* use and *not* for the benefit of providing advice or recommendations to third parties. Western Schools devoids itself of any responsibility for adverse consequences resulting from the failure to seek nursing, medical, or other professional advice. Western Schools further devoids itself of any responsibility for updating or revising any programs or publications presented, published, distributed, or sponsored by Western Schools unless otherwise agreed to as part of an individual purchase contract.

Products (including brand names) mentioned or pictured in Western School's courses are not endorsed by Western Schools, the American Nurses Credentialing Center (ANCC) or any state board.

ISBN: 978-1-57801-137-7

IMPORTANT: Read these instructions *BEFORE* proceeding!

Enclosed with your course book, you will find the FasTrax® answer sheet. Use this form to answer all the final exam questions that appear in this course book. If you are completing more than one course, be sure to write your answers on the appropriate answer sheet. Full instructions and complete grading details are printed on the FasTrax instruction sheet, also enclosed with your order. Please review them before starting. *If you are mailing your answer sheet(s) to Western Schools, we recommend you make a copy as a backup.*

ABOUT THIS COURSE

A Pretest is provided with each course to test your current knowledge base regarding the subject matter contained within this course. Your Final Exam is a multiple choice examination. **You will find the exam questions at the end of each chapter.**

In the event the course has less than 100 questions, leave the remaining answer boxes on the FasTrax answer sheet blank. **Use a <u>black</u> pen to fill in your answer sheet.**

A PASSING SCORE

You must score 70% or better in order to pass this course and receive your Certificate of Completion. Should you fail to achieve the required score, we will send you an additional FasTrax answer sheet so that you may make a second attempt to pass the course. Western Schools will allow you three chances to pass the same course...*at no extra charge!* After three failed attempts to pass the same course, your file will be closed.

RECORDING YOUR HOURS

Please monitor the time it takes to complete this course using the handy log sheet on the other side of this page. See below for transferring study hours to the course evaluation.

COURSE EVALUATIONS

In this course book, you will find a short evaluation about the course you are soon to complete. This information is vital to providing Western Schools with feedback on this course. The course evaluation answer section is in the lower right hand corner of the FasTrax answer sheet marked "Evaluation," with answers marked 1–22. Your answers are important to us; please take a few minutes to complete the evaluation.

On the back of the FasTrax instruction sheet, there is additional space to make any comments about the course, the school, and suggested new curriculum. Please mail the FasTrax instruction sheet, with your comments, back to Western Schools in the envelope provided with your course order.

TRANSFERRING STUDY TIME

Upon completion of the course, transfer the total study time from your log sheet to question 22 in the course evaluation. The answers will be in ranges; please choose the proper hour range that best represents your study time. You **MUST** log your study time under question 22 on the course evaluation.

EXTENSIONS

You have two (2) years from the date of enrollment to complete this course. A six (6) month extension may be purchased. If after 30 months from the original enrollment date you do not complete the course, *your file will be closed and no certificate can be issued.*

CHANGE OF ADDRESS?

In the event you have moved during the completion of this course, please call our student services department at 1-800-618-1670, and we will update your file.

A GUARANTEE TO WHICH YOU'LL GIVE HIGH HONORS

If any continuing education course fails to meet your expectations or if you are not satisfied in any manner, for any reason, you may return it for an exchange or a refund (less shipping and handling) within 30 days. Software, video, and audio courses must be returned unopened.

Thank you for enrolling at Western Schools!

WESTERN SCHOOLS
P.O. Box 1930
Brockton, MA 02303
(800) 438-8888
www.westernschools.com

Principles of Basic Trauma Nursing
2nd Edition

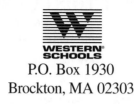

WESTERN® SCHOOLS

P.O. Box 1930
Brockton, MA 02303

Please use this log to total the number of hours you spend reading the text and taking the final examination.

Date	**Hours Spent**
_____	_____
_____	_____
_____	_____
_____	_____
_____	_____
_____	_____
_____	_____
_____	_____
_____	_____
_____	_____
_____	_____
_____	_____
_____	_____

TOTAL [ ]

Please log your study hours with submission of your final exam. To log your study time, fill in the appropriate circle under question 22 of the FasTrax® answer sheet under the "Evaluation" section.

Principles of Basic Trauma Nursing
2nd Edition

WESTERN SCHOOLS
CONTINUING EDUCATION EVALUATION

Instructions: Mark your answers to the following questions with a black pen on the "Evaluation" section of your FasTrax® answer sheet provided with this course. You should not return this sheet.

Please use the scale below to rate how well the course content met the educational objectives.

A	**Agree Strongly**	**C**	**Disagree Somewhat**
B	**Agree Somewhat**	**D**	**Disagree Strongly**

After completing this course I am able to

1. Describe the epidemiology of trauma and basic mechanisms of injury.

2. Identify the basic components of a trauma care system.

3. Describe the initial assessment of the trauma patient.

4. Describe the principles of shock management in the trauma patient.

5. Describe the principles of proper management of head injuries.

6. Recognize the causes and management of maxillofacial and neck trauma.

7. Indicate the major nursing strategies for managing thoracic trauma.

8. Describe the key components of managing abdominal trauma.

9. Relate the proper procedures for managing spinal injuries.

10. Identify the proper procedures for managing musculoskeletal trauma.

11. Describe the concepts important in the management of burn injuries.

12. Describe the principles of treating trauma in pregnancy.

13. Identify the important strategies in management of pediatric patients suffering traumatic injuries.

14. Apply the principles of trauma care for managing the acutely injured geriatric patient.

15. Identify the psychosocial issues affecting patients and families who have experienced a traumatic injury and also the staff caring for trauma patients.

16. The content of this course was relevant to the objectives.

17. This offering met my professional education needs.

18. The objectives met the overall purpose/goal of the course.

19. The course was generally well-written and the subject matter explained thoroughly. (If no, please explain why on the back of the FasTrax instruction sheet.)

20. The content of this course was appropriate for home study.

21. The final examination was well-written and at an appropriate level for the content of the course.

22. **PLEASE LOG YOUR STUDY HOURS WITH SUBMISSION OF YOUR FINAL EXAM.**
    Please choose which best represents the total study hours it took to complete this 30-hour course.

    A. Less than 25 hours

    B. 25–28 hours

    C. 29–32 hours

    D. Greater than 32 hours

CONTENTS

FIGURES AND TABLES

PRETEST

1. Begin this course by taking the pretest. Circle the answers to the questions on this page, or write the answers on a separate sheet of paper. Do not log answers to the pretest questions on the FasTrax test sheet included with the course.

2. Compare your answers to the PRETEST KEY located in the back of the book. The pretest answer key indicates the course chapter where the content of that question is discussed. Make note of the questions you missed, so that you can focus on those areas as you complete the course.

3. Complete the course by reading each chapter and completing the exam questions at the end of each chapter. Answers to these exam questions should be logged on the FasTrax test sheet included with the course.

1. Trauma is best characterized as

   a. the primary cause of death in the first 45 years of life.

   b. always requiring treatment at a trauma center.

   c. disproportionately affecting elderly people.

   d. a nonpreventable disease.

2. Hyperextension injury of the neck is most often caused by which motor vehicle crash (MVC) impact?

   a. Side impact

   b. Frontal impact

   c. Rear impact

   d. Rollover impact

3. Which of the following statements regarding trauma and injury prevention is true?

   a. Trauma is a disease of the underprivileged.

   b. Trauma is predictable.

   c. Trauma occurs by random chance.

   d. Trauma is not preventable.

4. Esophageal intubation can be identified by which of the following?

   a. Ability to talk

   b. Decreased breath sounds on the right

   c. Decreased bowel sounds

   d. Symmetrical chest wall expansion

5. A 50-year-old female is injured in a MVC, suffers a closed head injury, multiple left rib fractures, and bilateral femur fractures. She is orally intubated without difficulty. Initially, she could easily be ventilated, however the situation becomes increasingly difficult. Her pulse oximetry decreases down to 89%. What is the most appropriate next step?

   a. Obtain a stat blood gas.

   b. Auscultate the patient's chest.

   c. Perform needle decompression of the left chest.

   d. Obtain an x-ray.

6. A 40-year-old man sustains a gunshot wound (GSW) to the chest, losing an estimated 2 L of blood. You would expect

    a. his pulse pressure to widen.

    b. his systolic blood pressure to be decreased with a narrowed pulse pressure.

    c. his urinary output to be slightly lower than normal.

    d. him to be tachycardic but no change in systolic blood pressure.

7. The most common cause of hypotension following injury is

    a. hypoxia.

    b. head injury.

    c. blood loss.

    d. spinal cord injury.

8. In the head-injured patient, abnormally high intracranial pressure should be suspected when a patient exhibits

    a. bradycardia and hypotension.

    b. irregular pulse and narrow pulse pressure.

    c. tachycardia and hypertension.

    d. bradycardia and hypertension with a widened pulse pressure.

9. The most important assessment of a patient with potential brain injury is

    a. frequent neurologic examinations.

    b. frequent extraocular movement examinations.

    c. prompt computed tomography scanning.

    d. electroencephalogram monitoring.

10. With any head or neck injury the following assessment takes priority

    a. C spine x-rays.

    b. airway assessment.

    c. assessment for associated skull fracture.

    d. checking pupils immediately.

11. Retinal detachment occurs

    a. when there is a corneal laceration.

    b. primarily in elderly people.

    c. when the patient has a cerebrovascular accident.

    d. from various medical causes or trauma.

12. The first intervention to improve oxygenation after chest injury is

    a. intubate the patient.

    b. assess arterial blood gases.

    c. administer supplemental oxygen.

    d. prepare for chest tube insertion.

13. Flail chest is

    a. a serious contusion caused by trauma.

    b. a complication of pneumonia.

    c. when three or more ribs are broken, in two or more places.

    d. a result of extreme, harsh coughing.

14. Abdominal trauma

    a. is easily identified.

    b. can be overlooked because outward signs may not be present.

    c. occurs most often in children.

    d. occurs infrequently.

15. Which of the following situations would **NOT** create suspicion for abdominal organ injury?

    a. Stab wound just below right clavicle

    b. GSW to left flank

    c. Seat belt sign

    d. 11th and 12th rib fractures

16. The most frequent cause of spinal cord injury in young adult men is

    a. diving injuries.

    b. GSWs to the neck.

    c. falls.

    d. MVCs.

17. A 37-year-old male hunter sustains a fall out of a tree. He arrives to the emergency department confused but responding verbally. He is unable to move his legs. Vital signs are 80/60 mm Hg, pulse 64; respirations are 30 breaths/minute and shallow. He is on a backboard with O_2 by nonrebreather mask. Due to his injury the loss in intercostal muscle function will result in

    a. bradycardia.

    b. hypotension.

    c. inadequate ventilation.

    d. altered level of consciousness.

18. Posterior hip dislocation is a serious injury because it is

    a. an injury of elderly people.

    b. a common occurrence in MVCs.

    c. likely to impair blood supply to the femoral head.

    d. difficult to treat without surgery.

19. The "Rule of Nines" is a method used to

    a. determine the correct amount of IV fluid.

    b. assess the amount of burned body surface area.

    c. determine the depth of a burn.

    d. determine the depth of burns in each of nine body areas.

20. The most frequent obstetric trauma complication is

    a. premature labor.

    b. cardiac arrest.

    c. abruption placenta.

    d. uterine rupture.

21. Because a child's ribs are flexible, blunt trauma to the chest

    a. will splinter the ribs when they fracture.

    b. usually results in no injury.

    c. usually results in underlying pulmonary contusion instead of fractures.

    d. is an indicator of child abuse.

22. Priorities in the initial treatment of pediatric trauma are

    a. influenced by the presence of severe head injury.

    b. related to anatomic differences between children and adults.

    c. different if you are at a pediatric trauma center.

    d. the same as for adults.

23. Trauma in people over age 65

    a. is not likely to be any more serious than the same trauma in a younger person.

    b. is likely to be more serious than the same injury in a younger person.

    c. accounts for more than 50% of all trauma patients.

    d. is NOT related to elder abuse.

24. Mrs. Jones is pacing in the hall outside of the waiting room. Her husband was admitted 12 hours ago with a subdural hematoma sustained from a fall off a ladder. Which of the following has little influence on her ability to cope?

    a. Presence of close friends and family

    b. Previously developed coping skills

    c. The current presence and number of other stressors in her life

    d. Her education level

25. Which of the following best explains the gap between the number of organ donations and the number of people needing organs?

    a. The persistence of myths and lack of education on the topic.

    b. More people need tissues and organs than are dying.

    c. Medical care for transplantation is too expensive for the recipient.

    d. Clergy do not support it.

INTRODUCTION

Trauma is defined as any injury caused by a transfer of energy to the body. Trauma is a global problem. It is ranked as the third leading cause of death worldwide and the number one cause of death in the first 45 years of life in the United States (Moore, Feliciano, & Mattox, 2004). Trauma disproportionately affects the young and is therefore an enormous financial burden to society.

Trauma is often perceived by the public to occur suddenly and without warning as the result of random chance or an act of fate. Research, however, clearly reveals that trauma is highly predictable and is often associated with risk-taking behavior that can be prevented.

Trauma care is provided over a continuum. Injury prevention is the first phase of trauma care. Most trauma care centers and systems have an entire position related to injury prevention and working to educate the public on trauma prevention. First, the trauma patient encounters emergency medical services (EMS) who will stabilize and transport him or her to the hospital. EMS then hands the patient to the emergency department who will further resuscitate and stabilize the patient. If required, the patient will then move to the operating room, then on to the critical care unit, then the nursing unit, and finally to rehabilitation before being discharged.

Ideally, serious trauma is treated in a trauma center. Because there are only about 450 Level I and II trauma centers in the United States many patients are treated at nontrauma hospitals. Early stabilization and transport to a trauma center is highly recommended.

Trauma nurses work in many environments including prehospital, emergency department, operating room, anesthesia, critical care, floor, and rehabilitation. Trauma nursing is fun and exciting in the anticipation of the next unknown case. Trauma nursing works closely with other team members to assess and care for the patient. An organized and standardized approach is essential. Strong fundamental skills are requisite. These abilities critically affect the treatment and outcomes of injured patients, particularly in the first hour after the incident.

The purpose of this book is to provide a review of the fundamentals of trauma including the mechanisms of injury, common injuries seen, and resuscitation and management of those injuries. The level of information is basic and targeted to those nurses wanting an introduction to trauma care, as well as a review for nurses already working with trauma patients.

Course content includes basic concepts of trauma systems, triage, initial assessment of pediatric and adult trauma, shock, trauma to specific anatomic regions, burns and cold injuries, elder trauma, and the psychosocial aspects of trauma care.

CHAPTER 1

THE ETIOLOGY OF TRAUMA

CHAPTER OBJECTIVE

Upon completion of this chapter, the reader will be able to describe the epidemiology of trauma and basic mechanisms of injury.

LEARNING OBJECTIVES

Upon completion of this chapter, the reader should be able to

1. differentiate the years of life lost and cost between trauma, cancer, and heart disease.

2. recognize the common causes of trauma deaths in the United States.

3. specify the stages of the trimodal death distribution of trauma.

4. recognize basic mechanisms of injury and effects upon the body.

5. identify the impact of restraints and air bags in motor vehicle crashes (MVCs).

INTRODUCTION

Trauma occurs without warning and causes life-altering damage to the patient, the patient's family, and billions of dollars in lost annual productivity. Trauma is no accident and as such requires careful evaluation to assess the causes and contributing factors to develop a plan for prevention strategies.

FINANCIAL EFFECT OF INJURY

The cost of trauma care is overwhelming when viewed over the lifetime of a patient. Most trauma patients are young and many will become disabled leading to productive years of life lost. Figure 1-1 reveals how trauma is more costly than heart disease and cancer combined (McSwain & Frame, 2003). The economic impact to the nation is estimated to exceed $400 billion annually spent not only on medical care, but inclusive of dollars lost in wages, insurance administration costs, property damage, fire, and employer costs. Despite these monumental costs, less than 4 cents of each federal research dollar is spent on trauma research (Moore, Feliciano, & Mattox, 2004).

INJURY AS A PUBLIC HEALTH PROBLEM

Injury is the leading cause of death and disability among children and young adults in the United States. Trauma is the leading cause of death in persons between ages 1 and 44 and disproportionately affects the young. Figure 1-2 reveals how more years of life are lost to trauma than cancer and cardiovascular disease combined (McSwain & Frame, 2003).

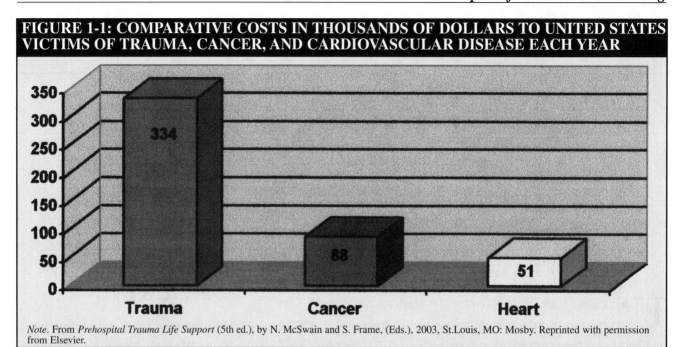

FIGURE 1-1: COMPARATIVE COSTS IN THOUSANDS OF DOLLARS TO UNITED STATES VICTIMS OF TRAUMA, CANCER, AND CARDIOVASCULAR DISEASE EACH YEAR

Note. From *Prehospital Trauma Life Support* (5th ed.), by N. McSwain and S. Frame, (Eds.), 2003, St.Louis, MO: Mosby. Reprinted with permission from Elsevier.

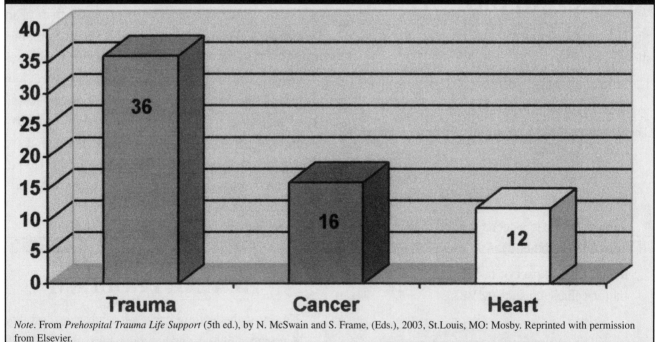

FIGURE 1-2: COMPARATIVE NUMBER OF YEARS OF LIFE LOST AS A RESULT OF TRAUMA, CANCER, AND CARDIOVASCULAR DISEASE

Note. From *Prehospital Trauma Life Support* (5th ed.), by N. McSwain and S. Frame, (Eds.), 2003, St.Louis, MO: Mosby. Reprinted with permission from Elsevier.

WORLDWIDE INCIDENCE AND SEVERITY

Unintentional injury is anticipated to become the third leading cause of death in all age groups by 2020 for the entire world. Injury does not discriminate based on age, race, sex, or economic status. It is the leading cause of death in persons ages 1 to 44 in most developed countries and is assuming a more prominent position in lower-income nations as infectious diseases are eradicated (Moore et al., 2004). MVCs account for the majority of injuries and deaths worldwide. Firearms remain an extremely lethal mechanism of injury. Deaths resulting from firearms are a particular problem in the United States. The availability of guns in the United States compared to other nations is felt to be a contributing factor to this problem.

TRAUMA AND THE U.S. HEALTH CARE SYSTEM

Over 60 million injuries occur in the United States each year, resulting in an average of 37 million emergency department visits. It is estimated that 40% of all emergency department visits are related to trauma of which over half are pediatric. For every injury death it is estimated that there are approximately 19 hospital admissions, 233 emergency department visits, and 450 office-based doctor visits for care for injuries (McSwain & Frame, 2003). Yet the rate of permanent disability to mortality is 3 to 1 (see Table 1-1).

TABLE 1-1: U.S. TRAUMA HEALTH CARE ENCOUNTERS
TRAUMA
For Every 1 Death:
• 3 Permanently Disabled
• 19 Hospitalized Admissions
• 233 Emergency Department Visits
• 450 Office or Outpatient Doctor Visits

TRAUMA DEATHS

Injuries are typically classified as intentional (suicide or homicide) or unintentional (MVCs or falls). Currently, violence and unintentional trauma cause more deaths annually in the United States than all other diseases combined. Violence accounts for over one third of these deaths. Motor vehicles and firearms are involved in more than one half of all trauma deaths, most of which are preventable.

NATIONAL TRAUMA DATA BANK

The 2004 annual report of the National Trauma Data Bank (NTDB) is an analysis of the largest aggregation of trauma data collected from trauma centers ever assembled. It provides the most compelling overview of trauma in the United States. Figure 1-3 shows the frequency of trauma by mechanism of injury and ranks MVCs first, followed by falls, then other transportation injuries, such as motorcyclist and pedestrian, and then firearms and stabbings. Figure 1-4 ranks the most lethal mechanism of injuries as motor vehicle crashes, followed by firearms and falls.

FIGURE 1-3: PATIENTS BY MECHANISM OF INJURY

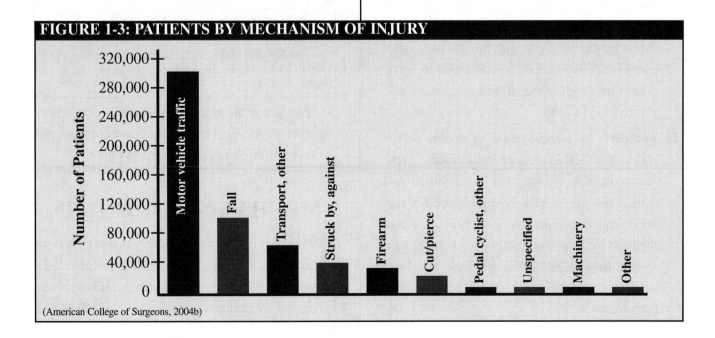

(American College of Surgeons, 2004b)

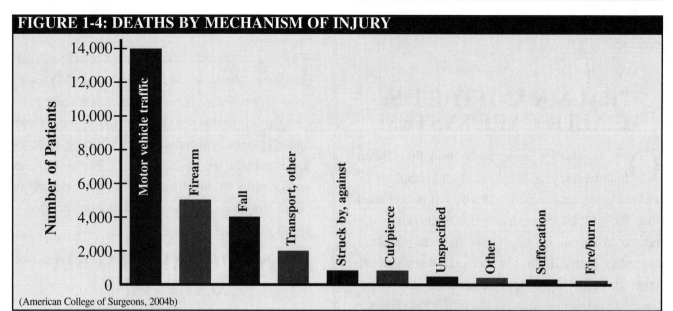

FIGURE 1-4: DEATHS BY MECHANISM OF INJURY

(American College of Surgeons, 2004b)

WHEN TRAUMA PATIENTS DIE

The Trimodal Death Distribution of Trauma

Figure 1-5 reveals how trauma deaths can be categorized into three phases. Fifty percent of deaths occur immediately at the scene followed by 30%, which occur within the first 4 hours. Finally, 20% occur weeks later during hospitalization due to multisystem organ failure (McSwain & Frame, 2003).

1. *The immediate or first phase of deaths* occurs within the first few minutes up to an hour after injury. These deaths likely would occur even with immediately available medical care and can only be affected with injury prevention measures. They include injuries such as aortic dissection, high cervical spine injuries, and severe head injuries.

2. *The early or second phase of deaths* occurs within the first 4 hours of the incident. These deaths include injuries that, if identified and treated quickly, would have a chance for survival and therefore are preventable. These injuries include pneumothorax, hemothorax, splenic lacerations, liver lacerations, and focal head injuries, such as epidural and subdural hematomas.

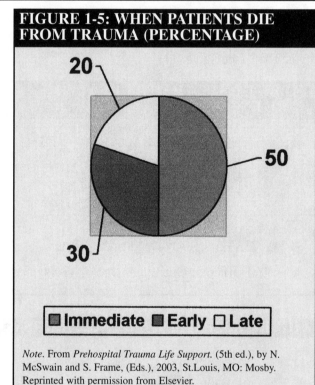

FIGURE 1-5: WHEN PATIENTS DIE FROM TRAUMA (PERCENTAGE)

■ **Immediate** ■ **Early** □ **Late**

Note. From *Prehospital Trauma Life Support.* (5th ed.), by N. McSwain and S. Frame, (Eds.), 2003, St.Louis, MO: Mosby. Reprinted with permission from Elsevier.

3. *The late or third phase of death* occurs weeks after injury, typically in the intensive care unit from multiple organ failure and sepsis.

MECHANISM OF INJURY

Trauma is defined as any injury that results from transfer of energy to the body (see Table 1-2). Exposure to different types of energy, such as kinetic (caused by crashes, falls, and bullets), chemical,

TABLE 1-2: ENERGY TRANSFER AND MECHANISM OF INJURY

Energy Transfer	Mechanism of Injury
Kinetic energy (KE) $\dfrac{KE = mass \times velocity^2}{2}$	Motor vehicle crashes Falls Pedestrian injuries Bicycle crashes Motorcycle crashes Assaults Firearms
Thermal energy	Fire
Chemical energy	Chemical substances
Electrical energy	Lightning Exposure to electricity
Radiant energy	Exposure to sun rays
Oxygen deprivation	Drowning Asphyxiation

thermal, electrical, or radiant, result in injury. Injury also results from a lack of essential agents, such as oxygen (e.g., drowning) and heat (e.g., frostbite). The injury occurs because of the body's inability to tolerate exposure to the excessive acute energy transfers. As a vehicle strikes another car, the crashing vehicle and its occupants absorbs the energy transfer. This kinetic energy is transformed into shock waves that the body's tissues must absorb.

Kinetic energy transfer is expressed by the equation mass times velocity squared divided by two. This indicates that in a crash, velocity carries more significance than the weight of the vehicle involved. Speeds of greater than 40 mph for unrestrained occupants predictably results in injury. With increasing restraint and air bag use, crashes of up to 60 mph are seen without predictable injury occurring. Kinetic energy transfers are the most common cause of trauma and will be emphasized throughout this text. Patterns of injury are related to the type of impact the driver or passenger sustained. Effects of an injury are also dependent on personal

and environmental factors such as age, sex, nutrition, premorbid conditions, and geographic considerations (rural versus urban).

OVERVIEW OF KINETIC ENERGY TRANSFERS IN TRAUMA

MOTOR VEHICLE CRASHES

Three Phases of Collision

Vehicular collisions are further subdivided into 3 phases (see Figure 1-6).

1. The car collides with another car or object.

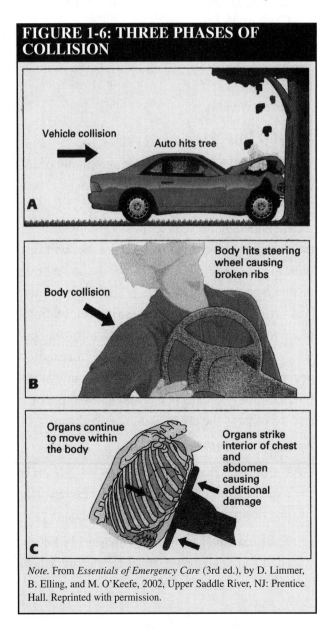

FIGURE 1-6: THREE PHASES OF COLLISION

Note. From *Essentials of Emergency Care* (3rd ed.), by D. Limmer, B. Elling, and M. O'Keefe, 2002, Upper Saddle River, NJ: Prentice Hall. Reprinted with permission.

2. The unrestrained occupant collides with the interior of the vehicle. The restrained occupant rides down the energy transfer belted into the vehicle.

3. The third collision occurs between the patient's internal organs and the external framework of the body (i.e., heart compressed between the sternum and spine).

Vehicular collisions can be categorized into the following types of impacts. Associated mortality rates are based on the total number of all fatal collisions as reported in the US Department of Transportation, National Highway Traffic Safety Administration's early edition of Traffic Safety Facts, 2004.

Collision type	Fatality (%)
Front impact	54%
Side impact	27%
Rear impact	5%
Rollover	9%
Unknown/Other	5%

Frontal Impact

Frontal impacts are the most commonly occurring fatal crash. In a frontal collision, such as a "head on" or "off set" (also called a "10 or 2 o'clock" crash), although the vehicle slows or stops abruptly, the occupant, depending on restraint use, will continue to move and will follow either the up-and-over or down-and-under pathway. If the crash is more "off set," the head commonly strikes the A-frame pillar that separates the windshield from the side window causing head injury. Figure 1-7 reveals how occupants in a frontal impact can travel in two different pathways. One is the up-and-over pathway and the other is the down-and-under pathway.

Up-and-Over Pathway

• Unrestrained occupants may follow a path in which the body's forward motion carries it up and over the steering wheel or dashboard.

• The head usually strikes the windshield while the chest and/or abdomen strikes the steering wheel.

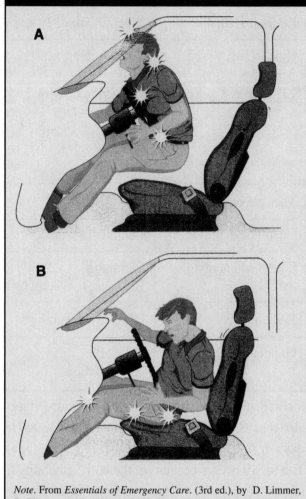

FIGURE 1-7: UP-AND-OVER PATHWAY & DOWN-AND-UNDER PATHWAY

Note. From *Essentials of Emergency Care.* (3rd ed.), by D. Limmer, B. Elling, and M. O'Keefe, 2002, Upper Saddle River, NJ: Prentice Hall. Reprinted with permission.

Down-and-Under Pathway

• Occupants who follow a down-and-under pathway move downward into the seat and forward.

• The lower extremities will be the initial point of impact with the knees or feet receiving the initial energy exchange.

• The continued forward motion of the torso onto the extremities may result in

  • Ankle dislocation

  • Knee dislocation

  • Femur fracture

  • Hip dislocation.

• The down-and-under pathway can be seen with restrained occupants as well.

- As restraint has increased, there has been an increase in the number of survivors of major crashes who previously were dead on arrival. With this increased survival, there has been a corresponding increase in severe lower orthopedic injuries noted that corresponds to the down-and-under pathway movement.

Side Impact

Side-impact collisions occur when a vehicle is struck on the side (see Figure 1-8). Side-impact collisions, while occuring less frequently than frontal crashes, are more deadly. The mortality rate of side-impact collisions is approximately double that of head on collisions. It is important to further define the lateral impact relative to the position of the occupant in the car, for example, being struck on the near side or far side. Restraint use in side impact collision has minimal protection, as there is only about 12 in. (30 cm) between your body, the car door, and the intrusion of the other vehicle. Newer side-impact air bags are beginning to decrease injuries in side-impact crashes. Statistically, lateral impact collisions occur more frequently in older adults due to their decreased ability to judge oncoming speed and distance of cars.

Four body regions can sustain injury in a lateral impact collision:

- **Neck.** The torso may move out from under the head causing lateral flexion and rotation.

- **Head.** The head commonly impacts the frame of the door.

- **Chest.** Compression of the thoracic wall may result in rib fractures, pulmonary contusion, and shear injury to the aorta.

- **Abdomen/Pelvis.** Intrusion of the door may compress and fracture the pelvis. Those occupants struck on the driver's side are vulnerable to splenic injuries (left side) and those struck on the passenger side are more likely to receive an injury to the liver (right side).

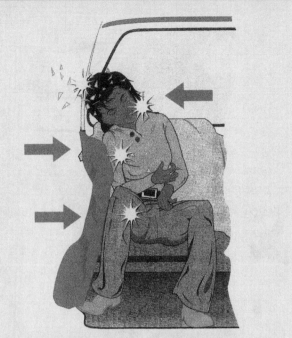

FIGURE 1-8: SIDE IMPACT CRASH

Note. From *Essentials of Emergency Care* (3rd ed.), by D. Limmer, B. Elling, and M. O'Keefe, 2002, Upper Saddle River, NJ: Prentice Hall. Reprinted with permission.

Rollover and Ejection

During a rollover, the vehicle sustains multiple impacts at different angles. If unrestrained, the victim will sustain injuries with each impact during the rollover and may also be ejected. Restrained victims however, often have minimal to no injuries in a rollover crash. Unrestrained victims incur the additional risk of ejection. Ejections from vehicles account for approximately 27% of all deaths from MVCs (US Department of Transportation, 2005). Clearly, seat belts save lives, just by simply keeping a person in the car.

Rear Impact

While rear-impact crashes are the most commonly occurring crash, they generally result in minor injuries. Rear-impact collisions occur when a vehicle moving at a higher rate of speed strikes from behind a slower moving car. Upon impact the vehicle in front is accelerated forward like a bullet discharged from a gun (see Figure 1-9). If the person in the car struck from behind does not have the headrest in position to keep the head in alignment

FIGURE 1-9: REAR-IMPACT CRASH

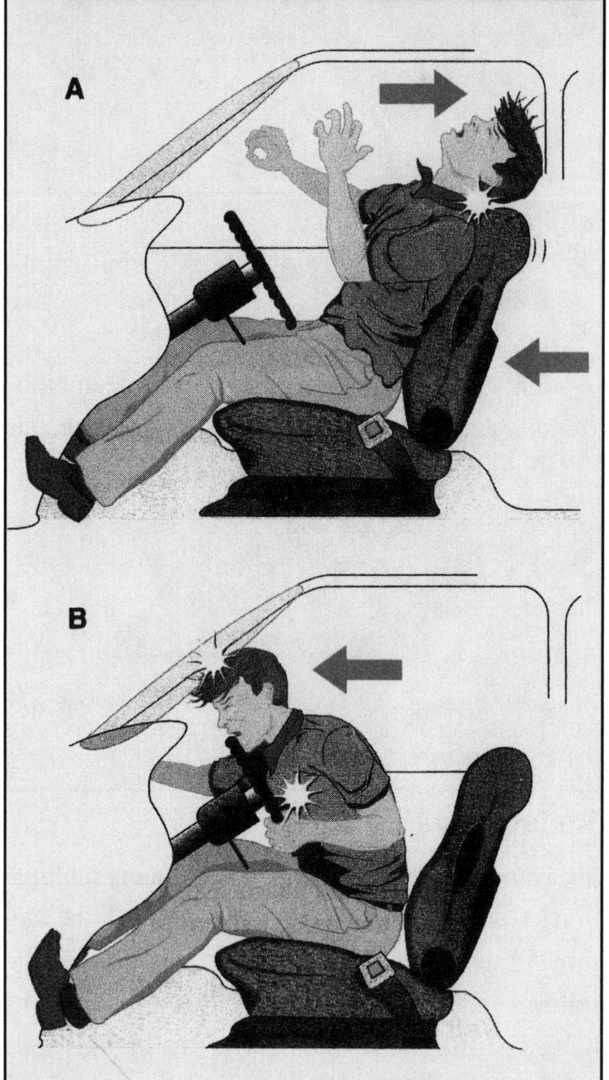

Note. From *Essentials of Emergency Care* (3rd ed.), by D. Limmer, B. Elling, and M. O'Keefe, 2002, Upper Saddle River, NJ: Prentice Hall. Reprinted with permission.

with the torso, then hyperextension of the neck occurs, resulting in neck injury. If the vehicle continues on to strike another car or the driver slams on the brake, a secondary frontal impact collision occurs as well.

Restraint Use

Restraint use in the United States has reached an all-time high of 82% (US Department of Transportation, 2005). Worn properly, seat belts anchor the body into the car and allow the pelvis and chest to absorb the pressure of the impact resulting in few, if any, injuries. When seat belts are worn loosely or are strapped above the anterior iliac crests of the

pelvis, compression injuries of the abdominal organs are known to occur. Lap belts should ideally not be worn alone. The diagonal shoulder strap should always be worn in addition to the lap belt to prevent extreme hyperflexion of the torso, which can cause injury to the lumbar spine and small intestine.

Air Bags

Air bags should always be used in conjunction with seat belts. They are not effective with unrestrained occupants and are only considered a secondary restraint system. They are highly effective in frontal or "off set" crashes. Because air bags deflate immediately after impact, they are not effective in multiple-impact collisions or rear-impact collisions.

Caution should be used with children and infants in cars with air bags. Children under age 12 should be positioned in the back seat. Never place a rear-facing infant car seat in the front seat, as the air bag will deploy directly into the back of the infant's head. Drivers need to keep at least 10 in. (25 cm) between themselves and the (steering wheel) air bag at all times. Short stature drivers should invest in pedal extenders to maintain an appropriate distance.

Motorcycle Crashes

Motorcycle crashes account for a significant number of motor vehicular deaths each year. They involve head on impacts, angular "side swipes," ejections, and the protective maneuver of "laying the bike down." In head-on collisions the driver travels up over the handlebars. In angular collisions, the driver is often caught and crushed between the motorcycle and the object struck. In ejections the driver is thrown from the motorcycle like a rocket. Once thrown from the motorcycle the driver is like a pedestrian, at risk of being hit again in traffic.

Motorcycle injuries are often varied in pattern making injury prediction difficult. When laying the bike down, the driver is taking a protective stance and turns the motorcycle sideways dragging his or her inside leg on the ground. This action slows down the driver and causes separation from the motorcycle.

Injuries sustained include friction burns known as "road rash" and minor fractures. Helmets have been shown to markedly decrease severe head injuries.

Pedestrian Injuries

More than 7,000 pedestrians are killed in the United States each year (Ferrera, Colucciello, Marx, Verdile, & Gibbs, 2001). Over 90% of pedestrian injuries occur at speeds less than 30 mph and the large percentage involve children. The variety of injuries seen are affected by the following triphasic impact:

- **1st: Bumper Impact.** Bumper height versus pedestrian height is an important factor in determining the specific injury. Adults are typically hit at the knee and thigh level. Children, on the other hand, will sustain more head, chest, and abdominal injuries.

- **2nd: Vehicular Hood and Windshield Impact.** Torso and head injuries occur as the victim is thrown up and onto the hood and windshield of the vehicle.

- **3rd: Ground Impact.** Head and spine injuries are common as the pedestrian finally falls to the ground.

Falls

Falls are the leading cause of nonfatal injury in the United States and the second leading cause of both brain and spinal cord injuries (Ferrera et al., 2001). Falls from a height greater than 20 feet are associated with significant injury. Landing position, head-first falls, feet-first or sideways falls, and type of surface encountered upon landing are all significant for suspicion for injuries. Head-first falls are obviously related to head and spine injuries. Feet-first falls are correlated with calcaneous, femur, and spine injuries, while with lateral impact falls the force is distributed over a much larger surface area and therefore has a decreased severity of injury.

Blast Injuries

Blast injuries are becoming more common with the increased threat of terrorism in the world. A blast explosion can be divided into three phases:

1. **Primary Blast Injury:** Primary blast injury refers to the wounding of air-filled viscera as a direct result of the blast wave. Eardrum perforation is common and serves as a marker of the proximity of the individual to the site of detonation. Primary blast injuries include pneumothorax, acute respiratory distress syndrome, air embolism, and perforated intestines.

2. **Secondary Blast Injury:** Secondary blast injury is penetrating trauma caused by fragments of bomb casing or projectiles.

3. **Tertiary Blast Injury:** Tertiary blast injury occurs when the victim becomes a missile and is thrown against an object. Injury will occur at the point of impact.

Penetrating Trauma

Low-Energy Weapons: Stab Wounds

Low-energy weapons include knives or ice picks. These weapons produce damage only with their sharp points or cutting edges. Because they are low-energy weapons they are usually associated with less severe trauma than high-energy, penetrating weapons. Injury can often be predicted by tracing the path of the weapon into the body. It is important to try to ascertain the length of the knife used. Remember that the entrance wound may be small but the internal damage can be great.

High-Energy Weapons: Firearms

High-energy weapons include handguns and rifles. In general, damage is caused not only to the tissue directly in the path of the bullet but also the tissue on each side of the bullet's path. The variables of profile, tumble, fragmentation, and cavitation influence the extent and direction of the injury.

- **Profile:** describes an object's initial size at the time of impact.

- **Tumble:** describes whether the object tumbles and assumes different angles after it enters the body.

- **Fragmentation:** refers to the breaking up of the object as it enters the body producing multiple smaller objects causing even further damage.

- **Cavitation:** high velocity bullets not only create a permanent tract but produce a much larger temporary cavity. This temporary cavity expands well beyond the limits of the actual bullet track and damages and injures a wider area than is initially apparent.

Entrance and Exit Wounds

Knowledge of the victim's position and the attackers position and the weapon used is helpful in determining the path of injury. It can be useful to determine whether the wound is an entrance or exit wound. An entrance wound is typically a round or oval wound with a surrounding 1- to 2-mm blackened area of burn or abrasion at the periphery of the wound caused by the spinning bullet passing through the skin. Exit wounds on the other hand are usually ragged or irregular as the result of tissue tearing. When examining a patient with two penetrating wounds it may indicate either two separate gunshot wound entrances with no exits or it could be one gunshot wound with both an entrance and an exit.

- **Caution:** Never assume that the bullet followed a linear path between the entrance and exit wound. Injury pattern is difficult to predict in penetrating trauma.

SUMMARY

In summary, it is important to know the basic mechanisms of injury and causes of trauma so one can have a high index of suspicion for specific injuries. It is helpful to understand the "big picture" of trauma's incidence and severity in the world, along with its impact on the health care delivery system. Understanding why and when trauma patients die, helps us to focus our care and where it is needed most.

EXAM QUESTIONS

CHAPTER 1
Questions 1-6

1. Trauma compared to heart disease and cancer

   a. is more common across all age groups.

   b. is less costly than heart disease and cancer combined.

   c. sustains more years of life lost than heart disease and cancer combined.

   d. disproportionately affects women.

2. Which of the following mechanisms of injury is the most frequent cause of death in the United States?

   a. Falls.

   b. Gun shot wounds.

   c. MVCs.

   d. Blast injuries.

3. The trimodal death distribution of trauma is characterized by which of the following statements?

   a. Most people die before arrival to the hospital.

   b. The largest groups of deaths occur in the intensive care unit.

   c. Early deaths in the emergency department are never treatable.

   d. Late effect deaths are frequently caused by cardiac disease.

4. Mechanisms of injury from MVCs are best characterized by which of the following statements?

   a. Trauma results from a transfer of energy.

   b. Car mass is more important then velocity.

   c. Injuries are predictably seen in an unrestrained passenger at speeds as low as 30 mph.

   d. Injuries cannot be reliably predicted based on type of impact.

5. The use of seat belts is known to

   a. prevent injuries in side-impact crashes.

   b. increase survival in rollover crashes.

   c. cause abdominal injury if worn appropriately.

   d. prevent neck injuries in rear-impact crashes.

6. Secondary blast injury is associated with

   a. bomb casing fragments.

   b. blast wave.

   c. victim as a missile.

   d. burns.

CHAPTER 2

KEY COMPONENTS OF
A TRAUMA CARE SYSTEM

CHAPTER OBJECTIVE

Upon completion of this chapter, the reader will be able to identify the basic components of a trauma care system.

LEARNING OBJECTIVES

Upon completion of this chapter, the reader should be able to

1. differentiate the components of an inclusive trauma care system.

2. recognize effective injury prevention strategies.

3. choose appropriate bystander actions at the scene of a car crash.

4. identify key principles of scene triage performed by Emergency Medical Services (EMS).

5. compare and contrast care provided at the four levels of trauma care centers.

6. select the variables unique to rural trauma care.

INTRODUCTION

A formal trauma care system will produce a coordinated continuum of care encompassing all levels of injuries including minor injuries, which can be treated at local hospitals, to severe injuries requiring a trauma center (Figure 2-1). In general the number of injured patients is inversely propor-

tional to the severity of injury. The most severely injured patients represent only the "tip of the iceberg" known as trauma.

INCLUSIVE TRAUMA SYSTEM

An inclusive trauma system involves a number of components, all of which must work together to meet the needs of all patients regardless of severity of injury, geographic location, or population density (Figure 2-2).

THE TRAUMA CONTINUUM OF CARE

Trauma care ideally begins with injury prevention. Injury prevention is believed to be the only means available to affect the large number of deaths that occur immediately at the scene of injury. Bystanders and then EMS personnel provide the next level of care. EMS personnel deliver the trauma patient to the closest hospital via the emergency department. The patient may be stabilized and then transferred to a tertiary referral center or admitted to the hospital. From the emergency department, the severely injured patient may go to the operating room or interventional radiology suite, and then the intensive care unit (ICU) or directly to the ICU, followed by the surgical unit and, finally, rehabilitation

FIGURE 2-1: SCOPE OF A TRAUMA CARE SYSTEM

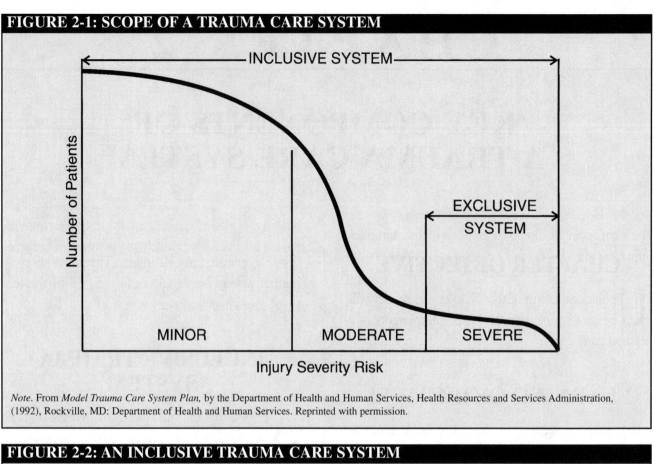

Note. From *Model Trauma Care System Plan,* by the Department of Health and Human Services, Health Resources and Services Administration, (1992), Rockville, MD: Department of Health and Human Services. Reprinted with permission.

FIGURE 2-2: AN INCLUSIVE TRAUMA CARE SYSTEM

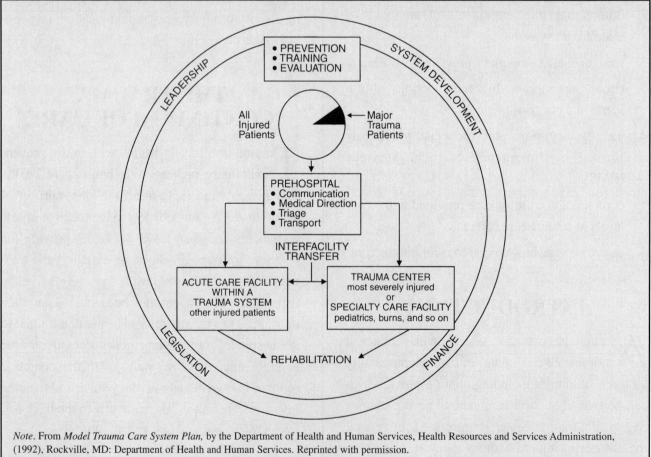

Note. From *Model Trauma Care System Plan,* by the Department of Health and Human Services, Health Resources and Services Administration, (1992), Rockville, MD: Department of Health and Human Services. Reprinted with permission.

if needed. Each phase in the continuum builds upon the other to provide optimal patient outcome.

Injury Prevention

Data collection and analysis leading to public awareness, education, community-based programs, and safety legislation are critical components leading to the primary prevention of injuries.

Trauma is no accident. Trauma is in fact highly predictable and can often be prevented. The use of the term accident should be avoided in that it implies injuries occur by chance or unknown causes. Most trauma deaths and injuries are preventable. The phrase "motor vehicle crash (MVC)" is now used in place of the phrase "motor vehicle accident" (MVA).

The trauma community has admittedly failed to capture the public's attention regarding injury prevention. The public has an increased awareness of cancer and cardiac disease risks but unfortunately not those related to trauma. Breast self-examination, blood pressure checks, and cholesterol screening permeate the public's consciousness, yet having 2 to 3 alcoholic drinks at a restaurant and then driving home without wearing a seat belt are commonplace behaviors. Trauma is often erroneously regarded as a social disease of the underprivileged and not an everyday risk to the general public.

The Three E's of Injury Prevention

Injury prevention is a scientific approach to identifying groups or populations of persons at high risk for injury and identifying strategies to eliminate or reduce the incidence of trauma. Most injury control strategies can be classified as one of the following measures.

1. Education

Education is the foundation of injury prevention efforts. Education efforts are aimed at the general public with the intention that knowledge supports a change in behavior. Although attractive in theory, it often yields disappointing results. Mothers Against Drunk Driving (MADD) is an example of an organ-ization that uses the education prevention strategy to great success. An informed and aroused public have led a crusade for tougher drunk driving laws that has resulted in a decrease of alcohol-related fatalities. However, for education to work it must be targeted to the specific audience, persistent, and linked to other approaches.

2. Enforcement

Enforcement is an effective injury prevention strategy. Education alone may impact some individuals to act but for many others the threat of enforcement is the only effective deterrent for risk-taking behavior. Different strategies work for different people. Seat belt laws are examples that resulted in significant increases in usage where educational programs alone had minimal effect.

3. Engineering

Engineering, while more expensive, often has the most lasting benefits. Engineering efforts however may have to be augmented with legislative initiatives for implementation on a large scale. The development and then legislative mandate requiring air bags is an example. Safety enhancements in highway design are another area of engineering effort that has resulted in increased safety while driving.

System Access

Rapid notification of an injury to the correct emergency response agency is vital to a favorable outcome for the trauma patient. One way this can be achieved is by providing *enhanced* 911 emergency services, which provides the location of the caller to the operator.

Bystander Care

You are driving along when you come across an accident with injuries that has just occurred. Perhaps you are the first, and maybe the only one, on the scene. The actions you take immediately can often mean the difference between life and death. The sooner a victim is treated, the greater the chance for survival. The first hour, termed the "Golden Hour," is critical in preventing serious injuries from turning into fatalities.

Simple life-saving steps recommended by the National Highway Traffic Safety Administration (NHTSA, 2000) as part of its National Standard Curriculum for Bystander Care include:

- **Decide to Help.** Stop, even if others are already assisting. "A helper always needs a helper." Do not fear legal problems if you do something wrong. Good Samaritan Laws in most states protect people from litigation should they stop and help as long as they act in good faith.

- **Call for Help.** While calling for help is important, assisting the seriously injured is more critical. If you are alone, provide life-saving procedures first, and call for help when all victims are breathing and major bleeding has been stopped. If more than one person is available, the more capable person(s) should provide medical attention while the other(s) summons help. Make sure whoever calls for help can tell the 911 dispatcher the exact location of the accident, the number of victims and their condition, and what help is being given. Make sure they stay on the line to answer all the dispatcher's questions and then follow instructions given.

- **Assess the Victims.** Check for consciousness. Is the victim able to answer you? Check for breathing. Gently tilt the person's head to its normal, eyes-front position and check for breathing. Hold your hand in front of the person's mouth and nose to see if you can feel breathing. Look for victims with head injuries (cracked windshield is an obvious sign) or who are paralyzed. If a person is talking or screaming, he or she is breathing. Move on to others who are not breathing. Look for victims thrown clear of the crashed vehicle or under the dashboard. Indications include an empty driver's seat, open doors, missing windshields, or an unoccupied infant seat.

- **Provide Life-Sustaining Care, if Needed.** Victims who are not breathing need your help first. Maintain an open airway. Remove items that might be blocking the airway, such as food or gum. If the person is not breathing, start rescue breathing. If available, cover the person's mouth with a CPR protective shield. Pinch the person's nose, if not covered by the shield. Blow air into the person's mouth—one breath every 5 seconds for adults and one breath every 4 seconds for children. If the chest does not rise, gently tilt the person's head back a little more. Continue rescue breathing until the victim can breathe without your help or professional assistance arrives and can take over for you. Once the victim is breathing, check for bleeding. Put on protective gloves, if available. Control bleeding by applying direct pressure to the wound using a gauze bandage or cloth. Wear protective gloves or use a towel or article of heavy clothing. If the person is able, instruct him or her to continue to apply pressure to the wound so you can tend to other victims or seek help. Stay with the victim until he or she is breathing and excessive bleeding is controlled.

- **Consider Your Safety and Other Responders.** Look for downed electrical wires, smoke and fire, the smell of gasoline, trees that might fall, or signs of hazardous materials. If too dangerous to stop, drive on to get help or get to a phone and call for help. Do not move victims. Never transport a victim in your vehicle. Put up warnings or have others warn other drivers of the accident without putting themselves in danger. Park your vehicles at a safe distance from the crash site and away from moving traffic with hazard blinker lights on. If you are first on the scene, raise your car's hood to signify a problem.

- **Develop a bystander kit.** Develop and keep a kit in your vehicle. This can be a complete kit, a basic kit, or anything in between. The simpler kit costs considerably less to assemble and could easily fit into a glove compartment while still providing most of the essential needs for bystander care. Typical kit items include a flashlight, gloves, gauze bandages, tape, airway mask for rescue breathing, towels, and blanket.

Prehospital Phase

Emergency medical service providers must:

1. Assess the mechanism of injury and patient injury status

2. Provide appropriate emergency treatment and determine the closest, ***most appropriate*** facility capable of caring for the specific type of injury (triage)

3. Transport the injured person as rapidly as possible.

Triage and transport guidelines are a vital part of a coordinated trauma care system. As a general rule, the order of priorities in multiple trauma victims is the same as in an individual patient where (A) airway takes priority over breathing (B) and circulation (C). Therefore, the patient with an airway problem is managed before a patient with a circulatory problem.

Principles of Triage

- **Degree of Life Threat Posed by the Injury**— always uses the ABCs of care to guide priorities.

- **Salvageability**—precedence should be given to those with the greatest likelihood of survival. A patient in full arrest on the trauma scene is most likely not able to survive and should be deferred treatment until others with life-threatening injuries are taken care of first.

- **Injury Severity**—treat the life-threatening injuries first. This is exemplified by the saying "Life over limb," which is an axiom that ranks life threats, such as obstructed airway or tension pneumothorax, above injuries to extremities, such as amputations or pulseless extremities.

- **Availability of Resources**—any patient whose needs exceed the local care available must be considered for prompt transfer to a higher level of care.

- **Produce the greatest number of survivors with the resources you have available.**

Stabilization and Transfer

When definitive care cannot be rendered at the local hospital, the patient requires transfer to a hospital that has the capabilities to care for that patient. Ideally the transferring hospital should be a verified trauma center. Research reveals that trauma patients have better outcomes when cared for in trauma centers. The patient should <u>no longer</u> be transferred to the closest appropriate hospital but should bypass local hospitals if access to a trauma center can be achieved within 30 minutes. Patient outcome is directly related to time from injury to properly delivered definitive care. Once the need for transfer is recognized, arrangements should be expedited and not delayed for unnecessary diagnostic procedures.

Acute Care

Trauma Centers

An inclusive trauma care system requires verification or designation of definitive trauma care facilities and confirmation of their commitment to certain standards of care, but **all** hospitals remain an integral part of the system.

Hospitals can apply to become a Level I-IV trauma center. However they must successfully pass a rigorous screening process held against high standards promulgated by the American College of Surgeons. A Level I trauma center provides the most comprehensive level of care while a Level IV trauma center provides minimal advanced life support care until transport to a higher level of care is possible (Table 2-1). Currently there are approximately 700 verified, designated, or functional trauma centers in the United States. These include 200 Level I trauma centers, 250 Level II trauma centers,

TABLE 2-1: TRAUMA CENTERS LEVEL OF CARE

Trauma Center Level	Care Provided
Level I	• Comprehensive trauma care • Education • Research • Leadership, outreach, and system planning • Immediate availability of staff and equipment • Minimum volume criteria of 1,200 admissions annually • Significant injury severity mandatory
Level II	• Comprehensive trauma care
Level III	• Prompt assessment, stabilization, and transfer to a Level I or II facility
Level IV	• Advanced trauma life support in remote areas • Resuscitation, stabilization, and transfer to closest higher level facility
Level V	• Designated in some rural states

and approximately 250 Level III trauma centers. (MacKenzie, 2003).

Rehabilitation

Rehabilitation is the process by which physical, sensory, and mental functional capacities are restored or redeveloped after damage. Rehabilitation has been shown to increase patient benefits, such as reduced length of hospital stays and improved functional outcomes. Appropriate and early rehabilitation enhances a survivor's potential to achieve maximal recovery, personal autonomy, vocational independence, and an independent lifestyle. Rehabilitation facilities are unavailable in many regions of the United States. Many rural trauma patients must travel hundreds of miles to access rehabilitation care, putting tremendous strain on a family's resources and endurance.

SYSTEM EVALUATION

A **trauma registry** is a computerized database used to evaluate the functioning of the trauma care system on a regional and statewide basis.

Trauma centers use the trauma registry for internal monitoring and processing improvement activities. It is also useful for prevention education, research, medical cost control, and improving patient care.

CASE STUDY

Without a trauma system. . .

At 10:00 a.m., a 911 emergency dispatcher receives a call that there has been a motor vehicle crash. Other than the location, no details are given and the phone call is terminated. The police are dispatched and arrive on the scene 5 minutes later. When the police arrive and realize the seriousness of the incident they radio for an ambulance. The ambulance arrives on the scene at 10:09 a.m. They find the patient unconscious, breathing shallow, but responsive to pain. They suspect internal injury and bleeding. The EMS providers notify the nearest hospital at 10:12 a.m. and relay vital information. The patient is finally removed from the vehicle at 10:20 a.m. and at 10:25 p.m. the ambulance is on the way to the nearest hospital. At that time the EMS providers are told by medical control to start IVs. At 10:35 a.m. the ambulance arrives at the hospital. After the physicians in the emergency room assess the patient, they realize the injuries are too severe to be treated at their facility. They call for a helicopter to transport the patient to a trauma center. At 11:00 a.m. the helicopter arrives and at 11:10 a.m. they are headed for the trauma center. One hour and 10 minutes have elapsed before the patient is on the way to receiving definitive care. This patient dies.

With a trauma system. . .

At 10:00 a.m., the 911 emergency dispatcher receives a call that there has been a motor vehicle crash. Because the general public has been educated on how to access the trauma system the caller gives important and vital information to the dispatcher who can then determine who should be dispatched to the scene. At 10:05 a.m. the police, ambulance, and fire department arrive on the scene. They find the patient unconscious, breathing shallow, but responsive to pain. They suspect internal injury and bleeding. The EMS providers radio the closest facility for medical help at 10:08 a.m. They are told to start IV's and to wait for a helicopter to arrive and transport the patient directly to the trauma center. The trauma center has been notified of the incoming patient and is prepared for the arrival. Meanwhile at 10:15 a.m. the patient has been removed from the car. The helicopter arrives and transports the patient to the trauma center arriving at 10:39 a.m. The patient is assessed and determined to need surgery. The operating room crew has been standing by and at 10:49 a.m. the patient is taken to surgery. This patient receives definitive care in 49 minutes, and is in serious but stable condition.

Check all of the issues in these scenarios that may impact survival:

- Bystander education
- Enhanced 911 capability
- EMS communication
- EMS trauma training

- EMS trauma triage protocols
- EMS trauma destination protocols
- Trauma transfer agreements between hospitals
- Helicopter activation protocols
- Trauma center activation
- Immediate availability of surgeons, staff, and equipment
- Immediate operating room availability
- ICU and rehabilitation care

Trauma is a time sensitive disease.

Triage Car Crash Case Study

You are the only nurse in the emergency department of a 40-bed community hospital. You have one doctor and a nurse's aide available to assist you. Ten minutes ago you were called and told that ambulances would be arriving with patients from an MVC. No other information is available. Minutes later, multiple ambulances arrive with five patients who were in a car traveling 60 mph before it crashed into a tree.

Directions: Triage and rank the patients in the priority that they should be treated by placing a number (#1 through #5, with #1 being your highest priority and #5 being your lowest priority) in the space provided before each patient case. The injured patients are as follows.

Patient A 50-year-old female was the unrestrained driver of the car who was thrown against the windshield. She is in severe respiratory distress. Prehospital personnel report the following suspected injuries: significant maxillofacial trauma with bleeding from nose and mouth, angulated deformity left forearm, abrasions to the chest. Vital signs: blood pressure (BP) 150/78 mm Hg, heart rate (HR) 125, respiratory rate (RR) 42, Glascow Coma Scale (GCS) score 8.

Patient B A 23-year-old male passenger apparently thrown from the front seat and found 30 feet from the car. On admission he is awake, alert, and complains of chest and abdominal pain. He complains of pain on any movement of his hips. Vital signs: BP 112/92 mm Hg, HR 140, RR 25.

Patient C A 42-year-old female occupant was found under the car. On admission she is extremely confused and responds slowly to verbal stimuli. Apparent injuries include multiple abrasions to the face, chest, and abdomen. Breath sounds are absent on the left and her abdomen is tender to palpation. Vital signs: BP 90/48 mm Hg, HR 142, RR 36, GCS score 10.

Patient D An 18-year-old female was extricated from the back seat of the vehicle. She is 8 months pregnant and complains of abdominal pain. Injuries include multiple abrasions to her face and anterior abdominal wall. You are told that her abdomen is tender to palpation. She is in active labor. Vital signs: BP 114/80 mm Hg, HR 102, and RR 24.

Patient E A 9-year-old boy was extricated from the floor of the back seat of the car. He was alert and talking at the scene. He now responds to painful stimuli only by crying out. Injuries include abrasions and an angulated deformity of the right lower leg. There is dried blood around his nose and mouth. Vital signs: BP 120/72 mm Hg, HR 182, RR 34.

Answers to Triage Case Study

Priority 1. Patient A.

Rationale: This female has a major upper airway obstruction. Airway is always the first priority in initial assessment of trauma. With bleeding from her mouth and nose, she is at high risk for fractures and swelling of the nasal and oral airways. Immediate assessment and intervention for airway should be undertaken.

Priority 2. Patient C.

Rationale: This female has absent breath sounds on one side along with hypotension, which makes her the second priority. The combination of these two signs and symptoms would make one suspi-

cious for a tension pneumothorax, which should be assessed for and treated promptly with a needle thoracostomy or chest tube insertion.

Priority 3. Patient E.

Rationale: This child has sustained a significant head injury as evidenced by his change in level of consciousness. Initial priority should be to secure and protect his airway. Early consideration should be given to transporting this patient to a trauma center with pediatric capability.

Priority 4. Patient B.

Rationale: This patient is stable and shows few signs of hemodynamic abnormality. The history of being thrown from the car, however, and the findings consistent with suspected pelvic fracture, puts this patient at risk for severe injury and possible hemorrhagic shock. He will need to be resuscitated and reevaluated frequently to watch for any signs or symptoms of deterioration.

Priority 5. Patient D.

Rationale: This patient is in active labor, possibly precipitated by the MVC. After examination and stabilization, care should turn to ensuring that there are no signs of fetal distress. Delivery is imminent, however this patient should wait until the other more critical patients are cared for first.

Rural Trauma Care

Seventy percent of the population of the United States lives in an urban environment, while 70% of trauma deaths occur in a rural locale. The chance of dying in a rural area from a severe injury sustained in a motor vehicle pedestrian collision is 3 to 4 times greater than in urban areas (Moore et al., 2004). The relative risk of a rural victim dying in a motor vehicle crash is 15 to 1 compared with the victim of an urban crash. In fact, death from MVC is inversely related to population density.

Trauma occurring in the rural setting presents a unique set of challenges not found in more populated areas. Risk of death is distinctly increased, probably as a result of prehospital factors, such as delayed recognition and inconsistency of EMS response and care. Many rural areas suffer from a lack of professionally trained EMS and instead rely heavily on trained volunteers. However, the lack of willing volunteers threatens the entire system and can lead to a severely disrupted response. Lack of trauma trained physicians and hospital resources also contribute to a higher death rate. Development and designation of rural trauma centers can be instrumental in reversing this trend. The education in trauma care that goes hand-in-hand with designation is probably most responsible for better outcomes of trauma patients. The guiding philosophy in such a system should be one of 'minimal acceptable care' with early recognition of major trauma and expeditious transfer of these patients. This does not obviate the responsibility of rural trauma centers to deal quickly and effectively with patients in whom ongoing blood loss is an immediate threat to life and to exert a damage control approach as an initial phase of treatment.

Rural Trauma Case Study

A 48-year-old banker was hunting with friends in a national forest in the Rocky Mountains. While separated from his friends he climbed a tree to survey the land. Seventy minutes later his companions found him unconscious at the bottom of a tree, after he had apparently fallen. One of the party rode out for help, which arrived in the form of a basic life support unit from the local ski area, approximately 1 hour after being found. The patient had to be extricated from the ravine and carried several hundred yards to the ambulance, which then drove 1 hour to the nearest hospital, a level III trauma center. Communication with the hospital was not possible until 15 minutes before arrival. His GCS score on the scene and in the emergency department was 8. He was hemodynamically normal, but a computed tomography (CT) scan of the head showed a large epidural hematoma with a greater than 5 mm shift; no other injuries were identified. Following consul-

tation with a neurosurgeon at the nearest level II center (150 miles away) a general surgeon trained in emergency limited craniotomy (and following established local protocols) drilled a burr hole and enlarged it sufficiently to permit evacuation of the clot and to control the hemorrhage. Poor weather grounded all helicopter transfer. The patient was transferred directly from the operating room to an ambulance, which drove him to the neurosurgeon for a formal craniotomy. He survived and is now independent, although no longer able to function in his former capacity.

What issues can you identify in the above case study that demonstrates the special considerations of rural trauma?

- Unaccompanied victim

- Hours or days to discovery

- Inaccessibility to rescuers

- Great distance to hospital

- Lack of trauma team and trained surgeon

- Adverse weather preventing air transport

SUMMARY

Trauma care should not be about luck. When you are injured in the United States you should be able to access an organized trauma care system that delivers the right care to the right patient at the right time. Everyone should work together to that aim. An inclusive system integrates all levels of trauma care in seamless delivery. We should expect no less.

EXAM QUESTIONS

CHAPTER 2
Questions 7-13

7. Inclusive trauma care is best characterized as

   a. all components of the trauma system are involved in patient care.

   b. only the sickest patients get treatment.

   c. there is only one trauma center allowed in the system.

   d. patient transfer agreements are not allowed.

8. The 3 E's of injury prevention refer to

   a. extrication, environment, encompassing areas.

   b. enforcement, emergency care, established protocols.

   c. environmental, emergency protocols, education.

   d. education, engineering, enforcement.

9. Which of the following actions is recommended for bystanders at the scene of a car crash?

   a. Avoid stopping for fear of lawsuits.

   b. Stop and call for help.

   c. Alert the local radio station.

   d. Stop traffic by stepping in the road and waving your arms.

10. Emergency Medical Services (EMS) provide critical services to the trauma patient. Which of the following are appropriate functions of EMS when called to the scene of a trauma patient?

    a. Insert an IV and then check for breathing.

    b. Check in with police before approaching the patient.

    c. Transport the patient slowly and carefully.

    d. Assess mechanism of injury and injury status.

11. Thirty-two patients are seriously injured in a bus accident on the local highway. You are a nurse working for a local trauma center and are part of a helicopter crew dispatched to the scene. Which of the following is a basic principle of triage?

    a. Treat the least severely injured patients first.

    b. Produce the greatest number of survivors based on available resources.

    c. Rapidly transport all patients to the nearest hospital.

    d. Treat the greatest number of patients in the shortest period of time.

12. Which of the following characteristics are matched to the appropriate level of trauma center?

    a. Level I trauma centers treat high volume and severity of injuries.

    b. Level II trauma centers are found in rural areas.

    c. Level III trauma centers perform research and education.

    d. Level IV trauma centers stabilize and provide rehabilitation.

13. Which of the following is a problem unique to rural trauma care?

    a. Short distances to the hospital

    b. Consistent EMS response and care

    c. Delayed recognition and inconsistent response and care

    d. Availability of emergency room physicians

CHAPTER 3

INITIAL ASSESSMENT
OF THE TRAUMA PATIENT

CHAPTER OBJECTIVE

Upon completion of this chapter, the reader will be able to describe the initial assessment of the trauma patient.

LEARNING OBJECTIVES

Upon completion of this chapter, the reader should be able to

1. select patients at high risk for clinical deterioration who require priority treatment.

2. differentiate the assessment steps performed in the primary versus the secondary assessment.

3. choose interventions to manage life-threatening conditions.

4. indicate the appropriate use of adjunct equipment or tests during the initial assessment.

INTRODUCTION

Initial assessment of the trauma patient is essential for recognizing life-threatening injuries and for determining priorities in care. It consists of two sections, the primary assessment and secondary assessment. The entire assessment should be completed within 2 to 5 minutes. It is an orderly, systematic approach to the patient to ensure identification of all injuries.

TRIAGE

The objective of triage (which means to sort) is to prioritize patients with a high likelihood of early clinical deterioration. A triage of trauma patients considers vital signs and prehospital clinical course, mechanism of injury, patient age, and known or suspected comorbid (preexisting) conditions. Clinical findings that stimulate clinicians to perform an accelerated workup include multiple injuries, extremes of age, evidence of severe neurologic injury, unstable vital signs, and preexisting cardiac or pulmonary disease.

When performing a triage of patients with several different types of injuries, the priorities of the primary survey help to determine precedence (e.g., a patient with an obstructed airway receives greater priority for initial attention than a relatively stable patient with a traumatic amputation). In trauma centers, a team of clinicians evaluates patients who are critically injured and simultaneously perform interventions and diagnostic procedures even while the assessment is going on. This simultaneous approach can dramatically reduce the time required to assess and stabilize a patient with multiple injuries.

The team approach to trauma is resource intensive; however, the available personnel and resources can become overwhelmed quickly in nonhospital settings, in smaller institutions, and in mass casualty situations. Under these conditions, additional factors affect the triage process, including the number and skill levels of available providers, the available equipment, and the provider's estimate of the probability of each patient's survival. The triage objective then becomes how to maximize the number of patients who are salvaged under the given conditions. This process can result in bypassing seriously injured patients until less critical patients have been stabilized. Triage under conditions of limited resources is difficult.

INITIAL ASSESSMENT

Initial assessment of the trauma patient should proceed in an orderly systematic way. The goal is to identify life-threatening conditions, identify injuries and to determine priorities of care. The initial assessment is divided into two phases, primary and secondary assessments (see Table 3-1).

The primary survey should be performed in 2 to 5 minutes. Simultaneous treatment of injuries can occur when more than one life-threatening state exists. The secondary assessment follows with a

TABLE 3-1: OVERVIEW OF THE INITIAL ASSESSMENT

Primary Assessment		Secondary Assessment	
Airway	Airway with simultaneous cervical spine immobilization. Can the patient talk? If obstructed, consider chin lift, jaw thrust, suction, oropharyngeal airway, and/or intubation, all while keeping the neck immobilized.	Head Face Neck	Inspect and palpate head, face, and neck. Check pupils. Assess GCS. Assess extraocular movements (EOMs). Inspect for jugular venous distention (JVD). Palpate cervical spine for tenderness.
Breathing	Assess breathing rate, depth, effort, accessory muscle use, symmetry of chest wall movement, bilateral breath sounds. Closure of any open wounds, oxygen, intubation, and ventilation as needed.	Chest	Inspect, auscultate, and palpate chest wall. Observe rise and fall. Assess accessory muscles. Palpate for subcutaneous emphysema.
Circulation	Palpate central and peripheral pulses. Assess level of consciousness. Look for obvious bleeding wounds. Check skin temperature and color in children.	Abdomen Pelvis Perineum	Inspect, auscultate, and palpate abdomen. Auscultate bowel sounds. Palpate for rigidity and tenderness. Palpate pelvis stability.
Disability	Rapid neurologic assessment Glasgow Coma Score • Best eye opening • Best verbal response • Best motor response	Extremities	Inspect and palpate. Compare right to left. Palpate pulses. Assess neurovascular status.
Exposure	Exposure, environmental control (Remove clothes, keep patient warm).	Posterior	Log roll patient. Inspect and palpate back and spine. Check rectal sphincter tone.

detailed slower examination. Next, each section of the primary survey will be explained in further detail.

Primary Assessment

Airway with Cervical Spine Control

While assessing and managing the patient's airway, care should be taken to prevent excessive movement of the cervical spine. The patient's head and neck should not be hyperextended, hyperflexed, or rotated to establish and maintain the airway. While holding the head, ask the patient to speak. This not only verifies patency of the airway but also will provide immediate information on level of consciousness. If the patient is unconscious, open the airway and inspect for foreign bodies, and facial, mandibular, or tracheal/laryngeal fractures, which may result in airway obstruction.

Observe for:

- Ability to speak
- Loose teeth or foreign objects
- Blood, vomit, or other secretions
- Edema
- Tongue obstructing the airway in the unconscious patient.

Interventions

Patent airway

- If the patient can speak, then the airway is patent.
- Maintain cervical spine immobilization.
- If the patient is awake and breathing and assumed a position that maximizes ability to breath, do not compromise this position.
- Signs of airway obstruction range from subtle to obvious (see Table 3-2).

Partially or Totally Obstructed Airway

- Logroll the patient onto his or her back while maintaining cervical spine stabilization.
- Remove any headgear to allow access to the airway. Patients wearing a motorcycle or sports

helmet who require airway management should have their head and neck held in a neutral position while the helmet is removed. This is a two-person procedure. One person provides in-line manual immobilization from below while the second person expands the helmet laterally and removes it from above.

- Keep the head in neutral position.
- Open the airway by either the jaw thrust or chin lift method:

Jaw Thrust

— Stand behind the patient's head and place the palm of your hands on either side of the patient's head.

— Place your thumbs over the cheekbones and position your fingers under the lower jaw displacing the mandible forward.

— Pull the mandible up using your thumbs as fulcrums to pull against.

— Using this method with mouth-to-face mask ventilation allows for a good seal with adequate ventilation.

Chin Lift

— Stand at the side of the patient.

— Place one hand on the patient's forehead to stabilize the head.

— Grasp the chin and lower lip with the other hand and lift the mandible.

- Reassess airway patency.

Suction: Anticipate Vomiting

- Be prepared for possible vomiting in all injured patients.
- The presence of gastric contents in the oropharynx confirms a significant risk of aspiration with the patient's next breath.
- Immediately logroll the patient onto his or her side and suction the airway with a rigid-type (tonsil tip) or (Yankauer) suction catheter. Patients with facial injuries may have associat-

TABLE 3-2: ASSESSMENT OF AIRWAY OBSTRUCTION

Method	Sign	Condition
Look	Tachypnea	A subtle but early sign of airway or ventilatory compromise
Look	Agitation	Suggests hypoxia
Look	Decreased level of consciousness	Suggests hypercarbia from hypoventilation
Look	Cyanosis • Nail beds • Circumoral (around mouth)	Suggests hypoxemia due to inadequate oxygenation
Listen	Noisy breathing	Suggest partially obstructed airway
Listen	Snoring, gurgling, crowing sounds (stridor)	Suggest partial occlusion of the pharynx or larynx
Listen	Hoarseness	Suggest laryngeal obstruction
Listen	Abusiveness or belligerence	Suggests hypoxia and/or head injury and should not be presumed to be from intoxication
Feel	Air from mouth	Suggests movement of air with expiratory effort
Feel	Trachea position	Deviation suggests tension pneumothorax
Feel	Midfacial fractures	Fractures of the mandible, especially bilateral, causing loss of normal muscle support and ability to protrude the tongue thereby obstructing the airway

ed cribriform plate fractures and the use of soft suction catheters through the nose should be avoided to prevent accidental insertion into the cranial vault.

• **Caution**: suction down the sides of the oral cavity being careful to avoid stimulating the gag reflex.

Airway Adjuncts

Nasopharyngeal Airway

— Used for patients who are partially responsive with an intact gag reflex. Ideal for inebriated patients who are sleeping off their inebriation or patients who are postictal, but to be avoided in patients with facial trauma, basilar skull fractures, or deviated septum.

— Select the largest size possible that will fit easily through the patient's nares. The size of the patient's little finger can be used as a rough guide.

— Lubricate the airway prior to insertion.

— Insert the airway with the beveled edge toward the septum.

— Direct the airway posteriorly and rotate it toward the ear until the flange rests against the nostril.

— Reassess airway patency.

Oropharyngeal Airway

— Used for patients who are unresponsive with no gag reflex and when intubation is not immediately available. Remember that the tongue in the unconscious patient is the number one cause of obstructed airway. Therefore this airway is inserted to keep the tongue off the back of the throat. It is a useful complement to bag-valve mask ventilation. In centers where intubation can take place promptly, oral pharyngeal airway placement is often skipped in favor of moving straight to intubation.

— Select the correct size by measuring from the tip of the earlobe to the corner of the mouth.

There are three methods of airway insertion:

• Method One (adult only): Insert the oral airway backwards, so its concavity (curve) is directed upward until it hits the roof of the mouth. Then rotate it 180 degrees so that the curve is directed downward over the back of the tongue. Be careful not to damage the teeth. This technique should not be used in children.

• Method Two: Use a tongue depressor to hold the tongue against the floor of the mouth and insert the airway with the curve of the tube following the natural curve of the airway. This is the preferred method of insertion for children and adults.

• Method Three: A hybrid of the above two methods, the oropharyngeal airway is turned sideways and inserted at the corner of the mouth and then rotated 90 degrees into position as the curve of the tube is advanced into the natural curve of the hypopharynx. This is an alternative method for use in adults.

• **Caution:** Regardless of insertion technique, always reassess the airway for patency after

oropharyngeal airway insertion to ensure that the tongue is not pushed down into the back of the throat.

Breathing

Airway patency alone does not assure ventilation. Adequate exchange of gases is mandatory to maximize oxygen transfer and carbon dioxide elimination. Breathing assessment uses the three senses of sight, hearing, and touch (see Table 3-3).

Oxygen Delivery Methods

Nonrebreather Mask

The nonrebreather mask is preferred for delivering the highest concentration of oxygen to a spontaneously breathing nonintubated patient. Nonrebreather masks with a reservoir bag with oxygen flow rates into the bag of 12 to 15 L/min. can provide up to 95% oxygen to the patient. This is the minimum recommended for all trauma patients requiring supplemental oxygen.

Bag-Valve Mask Ventilation

Bag-valve mask ventilation is required if the patient is not adequately ventilating. The bag-valve mask should have an oxygen reservoir and be connected to an oxygen source. Effective bag-valve mask ventilation requires a tight seal of the face mask along with adequate compression of the bag. The average delivered volume is about 800 cc. With a two-handed squeeze, over 1 L, can be delivered. Maintain an oxygen flow rate of 12 to 15 L/min. to keep the reservoir bag inflated.

Caution: Over compression of the reservoir bag is a common practice which can cause insufflation of air into the stomach, which increases the risk of regurgitation.

One-Person Bag-Valve Mask Ventilation: Stand at the patient's head and place the narrow end of the mask over the bridge of the patient's nose. Grasp the mask firmly with your thumb and first finger around the mask forming a "C" while spreading your remaining fingers around the mandible and

TABLE 3-3: BREATHING ASSESSMENT IN TRAUMA

Method	Sign	Implication
Look	Respiratory rate and depth	• Normal 12-20 per min • Less than 12 per min suggests CNS trauma • Greater than 24 per min suggests developing respiratory and systemic compromise associated with hypovolemia • Tachypnea (rapid shallow) • Assess for chest trauma, especially rib fractures, which cause pain and leads to rapid shallow ventilation and hypoxemia
Look	Abnormal breathing pattern	Cheyne Stokes (alternating pattern of hyperpnea and apnea) suggests possible intracranial injury.
Look	Diaphragmatic	Abdominal breathing suggests possible cervical cord injury.
Look	Accessory muscle use	• Bulging sternocliedomastoid muscle • Intercostal or sternal retractions • Nasal flaring in infants • Labored breathing should be regarded as an imminent threat to the patient's oxygenation
Look	Symmetrical chest movement	• Both sides should rise and fall equally. Always stand at the head or foot of the bed to view both sides of the chest simultaneously. • Asymmetry suggests splinting, or possible tension pneumothorax. • Paradoxical chest wall movement suggests flail chest.
Look	Skin color	This is a late sign and should not be relied upon.
Listen	Bilateral breath sounds	Decreased or absent breath sounds over one or both sides should alert you to the presence of thoracic trauma.
Feel	Chest wall	Assess chest wall integrity; inspect for abrasions, ecchymosis, penetrations; palpate for subcutaneous emphysema (crackling, popping sounds) or crepitus (fractured bone ends grinding).
Feel	Jugular veins	Bulging jugular veins suggests tension pneumothorax or cardiac tamponade.
Feel	Trachea position	Deviated trachea away from the side of injury suggests tension pneumothorax.

applying slight upward pressure. Compress the bag with the other hand. Alternatively, individuals with small hands may find it necessary to compress the bag against their body to adequately generate a large enough tidal volume.

Two-Person Bag-Valve Mask Ventilation: One person is at the patient's head and holds the mask in place with their thumbs on either side of the mask while pulling the mandible up slightly. The second person stands to the patient's side and compresses the bag with both hands to inflate the lungs. The two-person technique is ideally preferred whenever possible.

Temporary EMS Airway

Combitube

The combitube is used exclusively by EMS. It is commonly used as a back-up airway when oral intubation has failed. The combitube is a dual lumen tube that can be passed blindly into the esophagus or the trachea to allow bag-valve mask ventilation via ports from one lumen or the other. Most hospitals switch these out for regular orotracheal intubation after arrival in the emergency department.

Definitive Airway

Definitive airways include orotracheal intubation, nasotracheal intubation, laryngeal mask airway, and surgical airway. The need for a definitive airway in trauma is based on clinical findings of:

- Apnea

- Inability to maintain a patent airway by other means

- Protection of the lower airway from aspiration of blood or vomitus

- Impending or potential compromise of the airway like that seen in inhalation injury, facial fractures, or sustained seizure activity

- Closed-head injury or decreased level of consciousness as defined as a Glasgow Coma Score (GCS) below 9

- Failure to maintain adequate oxygenation by bag-valve mask ventilation.

The urgency of the situation and skills of the available provider dictate the specific route and method to be used. The potential for concomitant cervical spine injury is also of concern in the patient requiring an airway. Regardless of which intubation method is used, if endotracheal intubation is not accomplished within 30 sec. or in the same time required to hold your breath before exhaling, discontinue attempts, ventilate the patient with a bag-valve mask device, and try again.

Orotracheal Intubation

The nurse may assist with orotracheal intubation by helping assemble equipment, testing the cuff integrity with temporary inflation, maintaining cervical spine immobilization, and/or performing the Sellick maneuver (cricoid pressure with your fingers) during intubation to suppress vomiting and aid in visualization of the cords. Typical endotracheal tube sizes for women are 7.0 to 8.0 and 8.0 to 9.0 for men. The proper placement of the endotracheal tube must be carefully confirmed by the following techniques:

- Auscultate over the epigastric area first to confirm the absence of gurgling. If stomach gurgling is heard and chest wall expansion is not evident, inadvertent esophageal intubation should be assumed and the tube should be immediately removed.

- Look for symmetrical chest rise and fall.

- Listen for equal bilateral breath sounds at:

  - Second intercostal space, midclavicular line

  - Fifth intercostal space at anterior axillary line bilaterally

  - Equal bilateral breath sounds confirm proper tube placement.

- Use commercial end tidal CO_2 detector

- Once placement is confirmed, inflate the cuff, secure the tube, and continue ventilation.

Caution: Whenever the patient is moved, tube placement should be reassessed (see Table 3-4).

Rapid Sequence Intubation (RSI)

Intubation using pharmacologic agents has rapidly gained favor and is now the standard in trauma care (see Table 3-5). Rapid sequence intubation minimizes aspiration risk by administering induction and paralytic agents to the patient with a (presumed) full stomach. Indications for RSI include any patient who requires a secure airway and is difficult to intubate because of uncooperative behavior (as induced by hypoxia, traumatic brain injury,

TABLE 3-4: CONFIRMATION OF ENDOTRACHEAL TUBE PLACEMENT

Oral Endotracheal	Right Mainstem Intubation Tube Placement	Esophageal Placement
Absence of epigastric gurgling	Absence of epigastric gurgling	Epigastric gurgling
Presence of bilateral breath sounds	Presence of breath sounds on the right side only	Absent bilateral breath sounds
Condensation in the tube	Condensation in the tube	Gastric fluids in the tube
Bilateral chest wall expansion	Unilateral (right) chest wall expansion	No chest expansion Abdominal expansion
Normal oxygen saturation	Poor oxygen saturation	Absent oxygen saturation
Normal end tidal carbon dioxide detection	Normal end tidal carbon dioxide detection	Absent end tidal carbon dioxide detection
Inability to talk	Inability to talk	Phonation (ability to talk)
Chest x-ray helpful but cannot exclude esophageal intubation	Chest radiograph confirmation	Chest x-ray cannot confirm or exclude esophageal intubation
• Average female endotracheal tube insertion depth between 8.2 - 9.0 in. (21-23 cm) • Average male endotracheal tube insertion depth between 8.6 - 9.4 in. (22-24 cm)	Endotracheal tube insertion depth > 10.2 in. (26 cm)	Endotracheal tube insertion depth > 10.2 in. (26 cm)

hypotension, or intoxication). Rapid sequence intubation is not indicated if the patient is already unconscious.

Nasotracheal Intubation

Nasotracheal intubation has fallen out of favor and is rarely used today, but may be justified on the rare occasion when you cannot open the adult patient's mouth because of clenched jaws and you cannot ventilate by any other means. However, its application is limited to the breathing patient. It involves blind placement of the tube through the nose and then into the trachea.

Caution: Nasotracheal intubation is contraindicated in the apneic patient and whenever severe midfacial fractures or suspicion of a basilar skull fracture exist.

Laryngeal Mask Airway

Laryngeal mask airway is the insertion of a specially designed mask that is placed into the hypopharynx. It is used as a back-up device when endotracheal intubation is unsuccessful and effective bag-valve mask is difficult or impossible to do. Aspiration remains a possibility. If the gag reflex is present, a topical anesthetic or sedative is used to mute the response. The mask is lubricated and inserted with the opening facing the patient's tongue.

TABLE 3-5: SAMPLE PROTOCOL FOR RAPID SEQUENCE INTUBATION

Steps	Rationale
Ensure two patent IV lines, cardiac and pulse oximetry monitoring	• Patient monitoring for safety
Preoxygenate with 100% oxygen by nonrebreather mask for 3-5 min.	• Allows for 3-5 min. of apnea without significant desaturation
Pretreat with Lidocaine	• Reduces the cardiovascular response to intubation, used when increased intracranial pressure (ICP) is suspected • Reduces bronchospasm and airway reactivity following tracheal intubation
Pretreat with Atropine	• In pediatric intubation, prevention of bradycardia and excess secretions
Induction of sedation: • Midazolam (Versed) • Fentanyl (Sublimaze) • Etomidate	• Sedation
Chemical Paralysis: • Succinylcholine (Short duration) • Vecuronium (Intermediate duration)	• Muscle relaxation and paralysis • Used in the setting of suspected increased ICP • Used with open globe injuries to temporize the pressure rise during fasciculations
Sellick Maneuver (cricoid pressure)	• After administration of paralytic agents, used to decrease the potential for aspiration
Confirm tube placement immediately after intubation	• Continuous electrocardiogram and pulse oximeter monitoring is required during and after RSI
Repeat doses of paralytic agents as needed to maintain paralysis	• Use doses of long-acting paralytic agent, such as vecuronium, to continue paralysis. (Requirements vary with individual patients.)

The mask is pushed into the hypopharynx with the index finger until resistance is met which correlates with correct position at upper esophageal sphincter. A cuff is then inflated.

<u>Surgical Airway</u>

Inability to intubate the trachea is an indication for creating a surgical airway. Trauma conditions that dictate a surgical airway include edema of the glottis, fracture of the larynx, or severe oropharyn-geal hemorrhage obstructing the airway and an endotracheal tube cannot be placed through the cords. Methods for surgical airway include transtra-cheal jet insufflation and surgical cricothyroidotomy.

Tip: Please note that tracheostomy is not considered an emergency airway procedure. Tracheostomy is an elective procedure that should only be carried out in an operating room in a controlled setting. Emergency tracheostomy is discouraged because they are difficult to perform under duress, are often associated with profuse bleeding, and are too time consuming.

Transtracheal Jet Insufflation

Transtracheal jet insufflation is insertion of a needle through the cricothyroid membrane into the trachea. This is a useful technique in emergency situations to provide oxygen on a short-term basis until a definitive airway can be placed. It is also the procedure of choice in children under age 5 when endotracheal intubation is unsuccessful. Jet insuflation is a temporary "stopgap" measure allowing for up to 45 min. of extra time so that intubation can be accomplished on an urgent rather than an emergent basis. The jet insufflation technique is performed by placing a large-sized plastic cannula (angiocath), #12 or #14-gauge, through the cricothyroid membrane into the trachea below the level of the obstruction. The cannula is then connected to wall oxygen at 15 L/min. at 40 to 50 psi with a Y connector attached between the oxygen source and the plastic cannula. Intermittent insufflation, 1 s on and 4 s off, can then be achieved by placing the thumb over the open end of the Y connector on the side hole. During the 4 s that the oxygen is not being delivered under pressure, some exhalation occurs.

Caution: Carbon dioxide will slowly begin to accumulate and limits the use of this technique, especially in head-injured patients.

Surgical Cricothyroidotomy

Surgical cricothyroidotomy is performed by making a skin incision that extends through the circotyroid membrane. A curved hemostat may be inserted to dilate the opening and then a small endotracheal tube or tracheostomy tube, preferably 0.2 to 0.3 in. (5 to 7 mm) can be inserted.

Caution: Surgical cricothyroidotomy is not recommended for children under age 12 to avoid damaging the crinoid cartilage, which is the only circumferential support to the upper trachea.

Circulation

Circulation assessment in the primary survey involves rapid assessment of the injured patient's hemodynamic status. Key elements include level of consciousness, skin color, pulse, and evidence of bleeding.

Level of Consciousness

When blood volume is reduced, cerebral perfusion and level of consciousness will be impaired. Remember, however, that a conscious patient also may have lost a significant amount of blood.

Skin Color

Skin assessment can provide signs of inadequate organ perfusion such as pale skin, cool clammy skin, and delayed capillary refill. Ashen gray skin of the face and white skin of the extremities are ominous signs of hypovolemia. Any patient with pink skin, especially of the face and extremities, is unlikely to be hypovolemic.

Pulse

The patient's carotid and radial pulse should be evaluated simultaneously for presence and quality. A rough rule of thumb is that if the radial pulse is palpable, this provides an estimate of the systolic blood pressure to be at least 80 to 90 mm Hg. A radial pulse that is tachycardic and weak is an indication that the patient may be progressing into hemorrhagic shock. Unexplained tachycardia is indicative of hemorrhage until proven otherwise and should be quickly investigated. Hypovolemic shock should not be treated by vassopressors, steroids, or sodium bicarbonate.

Bleeding

Rapid external blood loss must be identified and managed with direct manual pressure. Internal hemorrhage should be suspected if hemodynamic status indicates hypovolemic compromise and there are no obvious signs of external hemorrhage. Major sites of blood loss include the thoracic and abdominal cavities, as well as major bones of the pelvis.

Reduce the pelvic volume in patients with displaced pelvic ring fractures by internally rotating the lower extremities and wrapping a sheet tightly around the pelvis or use a pelvic binder to do the same. Immobilize all fractures.

Resuscitation

Initiate two large bore #12 or #14-gauge IV catheters. Antecubital peripheral placement is preferred. All infused fluids should be warmed. *Adults:* crystalloid fluid bolus (lactated Ringer's solution, or normal saline solution), 2 L infused rapidly. *Children:* crystalloid fluid bolus 20 ml/kg infused rapidly. Administer blood products as needed: consider transfusion of type specific or emergency uncrossmatched blood: type O positive for men, type O negative for women. Prepare for surgical intervention if internal hemorrhage is identified. Monitor temperature and treat hypothermia aggressively.

Neurologic Evaluation

A rapid neurologic evaluation is performed at the end of the primary survey. This neurologic evaluation establishes the patient's level of consciousness and pupillary size and reaction. The GCS provides a quick, simple method for determining the level of consciousness (see Table 3-6). This is predictive of patient outcome especially the motor response. Remember that a decrease in level of consciousness may indicate any or all of the following:

- Cerebral injury
- Hypoxia
- Drugs
- Alcohol
- Hypoglycemia
- Postictal state
- Hypercarbia

Tip: All changes in level of consciousness should be assumed to be a head injury until proven otherwise.

TABLE 3-6: GLASGOW COMA SCORE

Eye Opening	4	Spontaneous
	3	To speech
	2	To pain
	1	None
Verbal Response	5	Oriented
	4	Confused conversation
	3	Inappropriate words
	2	Incomprehensible sounds
	1	None
Motor Response	6	Obeys commands
	5	Localizes
	4	Withdraws
	3	Abnormal flexion
	2	Abnormal extension
	1	None
Total Score		3 (minimum)-15 (maximum)

Exposure/Environmental Control

The patient should be completely undressed, sometimes cutting off the clothes to facilitate a thorough examination. Keep the patient warm with the use of warm blankets or forced warm air blankets. Monitor the patient's temperature.

History

Review the patient's past medical history for the following:

- Medications
- Allergies
- Past medical conditions
- Previous surgeries and hospital admissions
- Use of drugs or alcohol
- Smoking history
- Last menstrual period
- Last intake of food and fluids

Adjuncts to the Primary Survey

Pulse Oximetry

A pulse oximeter is a noninvasive photoelectric device that measures the arterial oxygen saturation and pulse rate in the peripheral circulation. It consists of a portable monitor and a sensing probe that clips onto the patient's finger, toes, or earlobe. Pulse oximetry is a noninvasive method to continuously measure oxygen saturation (O_2 sat) of arterial blood not the partial pressure of arterial oxygen (PaO_2). It provides useful information by its rough indirect relationship to partial pressure of oxygen (PaO_2). For example a saturation of 95% or greater by pulse oximetry correlates to an adequate, peripheral arterial oxygenation ($PaO_2 > 70$ mm Hg). The advantage of pulse oximetry is its ability to provide an immediate assessment of therapeutic interventions and detection of unsuspected hypoxia (see Table 3-7).

Caution: Remember pulse oximetry measures the percentage of (O_2 sat) not the (PaO_2). The hemoglobin molecule is so efficient at carrying oxygen that it is 90% saturated when the partial pressure of oxygen PO_2 is only 60 mm Hg (100 is normal). Therefore if you are used to thinking about PaO_2 (where 90 to 100 mm Hg is normal), then you may be fooled into thinking that a pulse oximetry reading of 90% is normal when it is actually critically low.

Caution: Many conditions interfere with pulse oximetry reliability (see Table 3-8).

End-Tidal CO₂ (Capnography)

Capnography, or end-tidal carbon dioxide ($ETCO_2$) measures the partial pressure of carbon dioxide (PCO_2) and when measured at end of exhalation it correlates closely to partial pressure of arterial carbon dioxide $PaCO_2$. It is useful because it provides a reliable means of confirming the position of the endotracheal tube in the trachea. In a patient being ventilated, the sensor is placed between the bag-valve mask or ventilator and the endotracheal tube. A normal end-tidal CO_2 reading in a critical trauma patient is between 30 to 40 mm Hg. As with all devices, there are certain conditions that will affect its reliability. These conditions include severe hypotension, high intrathoracic pressure, and any increase in dead space ventilation, such as with a pulmonary embolism.

Cardiac Monitor

The trauma patient should be placed on the cardiac monitor and observed for any dysrhythmias or excessive tachycardia.

Arterial Blood Gases

Arterial blood gases (ABGs) are useful with the sickest of trauma patients. Oxygenation and ventilation as well as tissue perfusion are assessed. ABGs will be discussed further in chapter 4, Shock.

Urinary Catheter

Urinary output is a sensitive indicator of the volume status of the patient. Urinary catheterization is contraindicated in patients whom urethral transec-

TABLE 3-7: PULSE OXIMETRY AND INTERVENTIONS

Pulse Oximeter Reading	Intervention
> 94%	Adequate, continue to maintain
< 93%	Cause for concern, assess for: • Airway patency, need for suction, oxygen, or assisted ventilation.
< 90%	Critical concern, immediate intervention required: • Open airway, suction, bag valve-mask ventilation, or proceed to intubation. • Assess for tension pneumothorax and prepare for decompression.

TABLE 3-8: CONDITIONS THAT IMPEDE PULSE OXIMETRY RELIABILITY

Condition	Rationale/Action
Poor peripheral perfusion, such as shock, vasoconstriction, and hypotension	• Avoid attaching sensor probe onto an injured extremity. • Try to avoid attaching the sensor probe onto the same arm that you are using to monitor blood pressure. • The pulse oximetry reading will go down while the blood pressure cuff is inflated.
Severe hypothermia (< 30°C)	• Inaccurate readings will result.
Carbon monoxide poisoning	• This will give falsely high readings because the sensing probe cannot distinguish between oxyhemoglobin and carboxyhemoglobin.
Profound anemia (hemoglobin < 5 g/dl)	• Inaccurate readings will result.
High ambient light	• High intensity lights, like operating room lights, placed directly over the sensing probe.
Nail polish or dirty fingernail	• Clean the nail with acetone before attaching the probe.
Excessive patient movement	• Probe dislodges easily affecting reading accuracy.

tion is suspected therefore a rectal examination should be performed prior to insertion of the Foley catheter. Urethral injury should be suspected if:

• there is blood at the penile meatus

• there is blood in the scrotum

• the prostate is high-riding or cannot be palpated

Gastric Catheter

A nasogastric tube is indicated to reduce stomach distention and decrease the risk of aspiration. Nasogastric tube placement is contraindicated when facial fractures such as a cribriform plate fractures are suspected. Orogastric tube placement is then preferred.

Radiologic Studies

The two primary x-rays ordered in all trauma resuscitations include the chest x-ray and pelvic x-ray. Cervical spine films remain controversial and are starting to fall out of favor due to a 10% miss

rate. Computed tomography (CT) of the cervical spine is increasingly utilized instead.

Caution: Transfer to definitive care should not be delayed by excessive radiologic procedures. Most trauma centers prefer to perform and interpret their own x-rays.

Need for Transfer

During the primary survey and resuscitation phase, the need for transfer to another facility should be considered early. Preexisting transfer agreements with trauma centers help speed the process.

Secondary Survey (Head-to-Toe Assessment)

Head and Face

Inspect and palpate the entire head and face for lacerations, contusions, and fractures. Reassess pupils and GCS score. Inspect for cerebrospinal fluid draining from the ears (otorrhea) and the nose (rhinorrhea). Inspect for periorbital ecchymosis (raccoon's eyes). Inspect for ecchymosis behind the ears (Battle's sign). Check for extraocular eye movements (EOMs) by asking the patient to follow your moving finger in six directions. Inspect mouth for evidence of bleeding, swelling, lacerations, and loose teeth.

Check for the Halo sign. Check for the presence of cerebrospinal fluid draining from nose or ear by allowing the drainage to drip onto a white cloth or barrier. A yellowish ring that develops in a circle around the drainage indicates cerebrospinal fluid. Do not pack the nose or ear or block the drainage.

Continue to maintain airway, ventilation, and oxygenation as indicated. Control any hemorrhage.

Neck

Inspect for abrasions, lacerations, or wounds. Inspect external jugular veins and use of accessory respiratory muscles. Palpate position of trachea.

Temporarily undue the cervical spine collar after cautioning the patient not to move his head or neck. Carefully palpate the back of the neck for tenderness and presence of "step-offs" (uneven or misaligned vertebrae). Resecure the collar when completed. Maintain continuous inline immobilization and protection of the cervical spine.

Chest

Inspect the chest wall for signs of injury (ecchymosis, abrasions, lacerations, punctures, or wounds). Assess for bilateral chest rise and fall. Check for use of accessory breathing muscle use. Auscultate the anterior chest wall and posterior bases for bilateral breath sounds and heart sounds. Palpate the entire chest wall for subcutaneous emphysema, tenderness, and crepitations.

Cover any open chest wound with a dry 4" x 4" gauze dressing taped on three sides only (flutter dressing).

Assist with needle decompression of the pleural space or insertion of a chest tube as indicated.

Abdomen

Inspect the abdomen and flanks for abrasions, lacerations, wounds, and old scars. Auscultate for the presence or absence of bowel sounds before palpating. Next, gently palpate the abdomen to determine the presence of rigidity or guarding. Always begin palpating in an area where the patient has not complained of pain or injury before proceeding on to the quadrant(s) with pain.

Assist with abdominal ultrasound, diagnostic peritoneal lavage, or abdominal CT as necessary. Prepare the patient for transfer to operating room, if indicated.

Perineum/Rectum/Vagina

Assess for the presence of contusions, hematomas, lacerations, urethral, vaginal, or rectal bleeding. Palpate for bony instability and tenderness. Palpate anal sphincter for presence or absence of tone.

Wrap a sheet around the pelvis or apply pelvic binder as indicated for pelvic fractures to reduce pelvic volume and control hemorrhage.

Extremities

Inspect upper and lower extremities for evidence of blunt or penetrating injury, including lacerations, contusion, and deformity. Palpate for tenderness or crepitations. Check all peripheral pulses for presence and quality. Assess and document all extremity movement.

Apply or readjust splints as indicated. Maintain immobilization of the thoracic and lumbar spine. Administer tetanus immunization as ordered.

Posterior

The patient should be logrolled to examine the posterior surfaces including palpation of the spine and rectal examination. The patient should remain immobilized until spine fractures have been excluded by radiologic and physical examination. Care however should be taken to prevent prolonged time on the backboard which can lead to skin breakdown and further complications. The patient should be removed from the spine board at this time if not already done by logrolling or the spine board should be padded if continued use is anticipated. It is recommended that the backboard is removed when the patient is rolled for examination of the posterior surface (Mikhail, 2002). The patient should continue to be log rolled as required until the spine is cleared.

PATIENT REEVALUATION

It cannot be stressed enough that reevaluating the patient frequently is necessary to avoid missing injuries. When vital signs suddenly deteriorate, one should immediately return to the primary survey and prepare to intervene. Many injuries are not apparent on first assessment and actually only become apparent over time. Distracting injuries, such as painful femur fractures, keep the patient from voicing other concerns that will become obvious only later. Verbal and nonverbal feedback of the patient during physical examination is helpful to identify suspected injuries. Therefore, judicious use of analgesics is recommended during the initial assessment to avoid masking the patient's response to physical examination. Continuous monitoring of the vital signs, urinary output, and pulse oximetry is essential as the patient can deteriorate at anytime. Nursing should remain vigilant and monitoring of the patient should continue until all injuries are identified.

SUMMARY

In summary, a rapid but thorough initial assessment is a vital skill for the trauma nurse to master. Early identification and intervention of life-threatening injuries is responsible for the decreasing early death rate noted among trauma patients who are treated at trauma centers across the United States. Utilizing a systematic assessment ensures that the patient's injuries will be identified and treat-

ed resulting in an optimal outcome with the least disability.

EXAM QUESTIONS

CHAPTER 3

Questions 14-22

14. You are the only registered nurse working in a small six-bed emergency department when multiple ambulances arrive with three patients from a single car motor vehicle crash. Triage the following patients to be treated first, second, and third.

    Patient 1: 22-year-old male who was the unrestrained driver of the car who was ejected. Admission respiratory rate noted of 42 with copious blood noted from nose and mouth with gurgling sounds. Angulated right arm and multiple abrasions noted to chest. Vitals: BP 145/82 mm Hg, HR 128, RR 44. GCS = 6.

    Patient 2: A 5-year-old female extricated from the backseat. She responds only to painful stimuli. Dried blood noted to nares. Vitals: BP 110/70 mm Hg, HR 180, RR 18. GCS = 6.

    Patient 3: A 20-year-old female passenger was found in the front seat. She is confused and responds slowly to verbal stimuli. Breath sounds are absent on the right. There is a superficial laceration to the right arm and abrasion noted to the legs and abdomen. Vitals: BP 90/58 mm Hg, HR 144, RR 20. GCS = 14.

    The patients should be treated in the following order

    a. 1, 2, 3
    b. 2, 1, 3
    c. 3, 2, 1
    d. 1, 3, 2

15. Which of the following findings in an adult trauma patient should prompt immediate return to the primary survey for assessment and intervention?

    a. Heart rate of 110
    b. GCS of 12
    c. Temperature of 36.5° C
    d. Respiratory rate of 40 breaths/min.

16. Which of the following procedures is performed in the primary assessment?

    a. Bowel sounds
    b. Pulse check
    c. Neurovascular extremity checks
    d. Rectal examination

17. During the initial assessment, the patient injured by a fall from 20 feet should be completely immobilized until

    a. the patient is able to indicate that he has no neck pain.
    b. the patient complains of potential pressure sores due to the board.
    c. a spinal fracture has been ruled out both by x-rays and examination.
    d. the full neurologic examination has been completed.

18. A 16-year-old female who was thrown from a horse arrives by private car to your emergency department. You are the only registered nurse on duty and the only emergency physician has left for a meeting. Assessment reveals a deteriorating mental status GCS = 6, ventilation 8 per min. with sonorous respirations and a strong radial pulse of 78 beats/min. Which is the most appropriate treatment at this time?

   a. Oropharyngeal airway placement and bag-valve mask ventilation

   b. Supplemental oxygen via nonrebreather mask at 12 to 15 L/min.

   c. Nasopharyngeal airway with nonrebreather mask at 15 liters per min.

   d. Mouth-to-mouth resuscitation.

19. A 17-year-old man, injured in an MVC, sustains a closed-head injury with a GCS of 8. His BP is 100/50 mm Hg, HR is 80, and RR is 22. He has a right femur fracture, a left humerus fracture, and multiple palpable rib fractures on the left side. Initially, his ventilation is easily assisted with a bag-valve device. It gradually becomes more difficult to ventilate and his blood pressure drops precipitously. His pulse oximetry drops from 97% to 88%. Which of the following is the most appropriate initial nursing action to take?

   a. Auscultate the patient's chest.

   b. Prepare for needle decompression of the left chest.

   c. Increase IVs to wide open.

   d. Order emergency uncrossmatched blood stat.

20. Rapid sequence intubation is indicated for

   a. unconscious patients.

   b. patients who are combative.

   c. alert patients with nasal fractures.

   d. inexperienced intubation personnel.

21. Pulse oximetry in trauma patients is best utilized as a

   a. measure of the patients PaO_2.

   b. measure of SaO_2 in severely hypothermic patients.

   c. noninvasive continuous measure of O_2 sat.

   d. means for alarm when it stays above 93%.

22. Nasogastric tube placement in trauma can

   a. increase the risk of aspiration.

   b. decrease gastric distention.

   c. provide nasal packing for nasal fractures.

   d. prevent drainage into the oropharyngeal airway.

CHAPTER 4

SHOCK

CHAPTER OBJECTIVE

Upon completion of this chapter, the reader will be able to describe the principles of shock management in the trauma patient.

LEARNING OBJECTIVES

Upon completion of this chapter the reader should be able to

1. define shock.

2. recognize the effects of compensatory mechanisms on vital signs.

3. discriminate between the four classes of hemorrhagic shock.

4. differentiate between the major types of shock.

5. recognize confounding factors in the trauma patient's response to hemorrhage.

6. choose appropriate nursing interventions to treat hemorrhagic shock.

7. identify current methods of prevention and treatment of hypothermia.

INTRODUCTION

Shock is a syndrome resulting from inadequate perfusion of the tissues. This inadequacy leads to a decrease in the supply of oxygen to the cells. The body responds to this situation with compensatory mechanisms to improve perfusion, especially in high-demand areas, such as the heart and brain. The nurse should be prepared to assess, identify, and intervene in shock states.

DEFINITION AND BASIC PHYSIOLOGY

Shock can be defined in two words: inadequate perfusion. There is a decrease in circulating blood volume (supply) or utilization of oxygen and nutrients by the cell. Remember that shock is a problem of decreased perfusion, not decreased blood pressure. It is inadequate perfusion of end organs, such as the brain, heart, lungs, and kidneys. The predominate physiologic deficit resulting from inadequate perfusion is metabolic acidosis. When tissue hypoxia is present, normal cell physiology is altered, and a shift from aerobic to anaerobic metabolism occurs, resulting in lactic acidosis. The negative effects of acidosis on the cardiovascular system include decreased cardiac contractility, decreased cardiac output, vasodilatation, and hypotension. The body responds initially by the use of compensatory mechanisms to improve perfusion. If the compensatory mechanisms fail to restore perfusion, then organ dysfunction and eventually cell death occur.

COMPENSATORY MECHANISMS OVERVIEW

As cardiac output decreases, the body responds with compensatory mechanisms. The decreased blood flow stimulates pressoreceptors located in the aorta and carotid bodies to send a message to the medulla in the brain thereby activating the sympathetic nervous system. Sympathetic nervous system activation shunts blood flow to the vital organs (the heart and the brain) and directs blood away from nonpriority organs such as the skin, gastrointestinal tract, and lungs. The response to volume depletion is an increase in heart rate in an attempt to preserve cardiac output. Tachycardia therefore is an early circulatory sign of shock. There is a release of endogenous catecholamines, epinephrine and norepinephrine, which increase peripheral vascular resistance. This release increases the diastolic blood pressure, and reduces pulse pressure, but does little to improve end-organ perfusion. Vasoconstriction causes the skin to become cool and clammy. The lungs increase the rate and depth of respirations. Decreased renal blood flow results in decreased urine output. These compensatory mechanisms are visible through the changes in the patient's vital signs (see Table 4-1).

Tip: Any patient who is cool and tachycardic is in shock until proven otherwise.

CLINICAL DIFFERENTIATION OF SHOCK

Shock in a trauma patient can be simply classified as hemorrhagic or nonhemorrhagic. Hemorrhagic shock is by far the most common form of shock after trauma. Careful consideration, however, should be given to rule out other nonhemorrhagic forms as well. These include cardiogenic, tension pneumothorax, neurogenic, and septic shock.

TABLE 4-1: ASSESSMENT OF VITAL SIGNS IN SHOCK	

Blood Pressure (BP)	• Late sign of inadequate perfusion
	• Systolic pressure does not drop until:
	   • 30% of blood volume lost in adults
	   • 40-45% in pediatrics
	• Initial BP confirmed manually in trauma patients before relying on automated BP machine assessment

Pulse Rate	• Erratic sign affected by pain, fever, drugs, and emotions • Tachycardia trended over time has value
Pulse Pressure	• Narrowed pulse pressure noted early in shock • Result of diastolic pressure rising, not systolic pressure falling
Respiratory Rate	• Increased rate and depth initially • Decreased rate and depth as shock progresses
Mentation	• Initially agitation and anxiousness noted in early shock • Progressive decreased level of consciousness as shock progresses • Rule out other causes: hypoxia, head injury, drugs, alcohol

CLASSIFICATION OF SHOCK

Cardiogenic Shock

Cardiogenic shock results from ineffective perfusion caused by decreased contractility of the heart. Cardiogenic shock is rarely seen following trauma but may occur following blunt cardiac injury, cardiac tamponade, and myocardial infarction. Blunt cardiac injury should be suspected when the mechanism of injury is rapid deceleration, such as in a high fall or motor vehicular crash. Continuous electrocardiograph monitoring is warranted to detect dysrhythmias. Echocardiography can be useful but is often difficult to obtain quickly. Cardiac tamponade is associated most commonly with penetrating trauma to the chest. Tachycardia, muffled heart tones, jugular venous distention, vasoconstriction, and hypotension are hallmarks of this injury. A quick ultrasound of the heart region known as Focused Assessment Sonography in Trauma (FAST) is helpful to quickly identify fluid in the pericardial sac. Treatment measures include needle pericardiocentesis followed by immediate transfer to the operating room for open cardiac window procedure.

Tension Pneumothorax

Tension Pneumothorax after injury occurs when air is allowed to enter the pleural space but is not allowed to escape. This causes intrapleural pressure to rise, resulting in a total lung collapse and a shift of the mediastinum to the opposite side with impairment of venous return and acute fall in cardiac output. The patient will present with acute respiratory distress, jugular venous distention, subcutaneous emphysema, absent breath sounds, hyperresonnance to percussion, and tracheal shift away from the side of injury. Immediate treatment with needle decompression is warranted without delaying for x-ray confirmation.

Neurogenic Shock

Neurogenic shock may occur as a result of injury to the spinal cord. Sympathetic nervous system function is impaired resulting in loss of vasomotor tone resulting in peripheral vasodilatation and maldistribution of blood volume causing hypotension. Corresponding increased parasympathetic tone can result in bradycardia. The classic picture of neurogenic shock is hypotension without tachycardia or cutaneous vasoconstriction. A narrowed pulse pressure is not seen in neurogenic shock. The blood pressure may not be restored by fluid administration alone. Cautious use of vassopressors after moderate fluid replacement may be justified. Atropine may be used to counteract hemodynamically significant bradycardia. Remember that patients with spinal cord injury often have concomitant chest and abdominal injuries. Therefore, patients with suspected neurogenic shock should initially be treated for hypovolemia. This is detailed further in chapter 9, Trauma to the Spine.

Septic Shock

Septic shock is not seen immediately after injury. It is a problem seen days and/or weeks later in the critical care unit. Septic patients who are hypotensive and afebrile are clinically difficult to distinguish from those in hypovolemic shock.

Patients in late septic shock may present with tachycardia, vasoconstriction, decreased urine output, decreased systolic pressure, and narrow pulse pressure. Early septic shock, however, is demonstrated with tachycardia, vasodilation, warm pink skin, a systolic pressure near normal, and a wide pulse pressure.

Hemorrhagic Shock

Hemorrhagic shock is caused by a decrease in the circulating blood volume. In general, it is important to remember that the primary focus is to identify and stop hemorrhage promptly in the trauma patient. This will be discussed in detail later in this chapter. Hemorrhagic shock can be further classified based on blood volume loss (see Table 4-2).

Class I

Class I involves a blood loss up to 750 ml. This is equivalent to donating a unit of blood. No measurable changes occur in blood pressure, pulse pressure, or respiratory rate. Hydration with oral fluids is all that is commonly necessary.

Class II

Class II represents a 750 to 1,500 ml blood loss. Symptoms typically include tachycardia, tachypnea, and decreased pulse pressure. The decrease in pulse pressure results from an increase in the diastolic pressure, not a drop in the systolic pressure. The patient may demonstrate anxiety or agitation, which may be symptomatic of decreased cerebral blood flow.

Class III

Class III involves a 1,500 to 2,000 ml blood loss. The patient presents with significant tachycardia, hypotension, tachypnea, and altered level of consciousness. It is important to stress that Class III hemorrhage occurs when you finally note a drop in systolic pressure. Typically the patient requires aggressive fluid resuscitation with blood replacement.

Class IV

Class IV is a blood loss greater than 2,000 ml or over 40% blood volume loss. This loss represents life-threatening hemorrhage with the patient presenting in extremis. Symptoms include extreme tachycardia, hypotension, narrowed pulse pressure, and/or undetectable diastolic pressure. The skin is cool and clammy. The urine output is negligible and there is marked depressed level of consciousness. Aggressive resuscitation and immediate surgery are required to turn this situation around quickly.

Confounding Factors in Trauma Patients' Response

Several factors affect trauma patients' response include age, athletic ability, pregnancy, and medications (see Table 4-3).

Sites of Blood Loss

The three main areas where blood loss is highly suspected in trauma are the chest, abdomen, and pelvis. Major soft tissue injuries and fractures however also can compromise hemodynamics as well.

TABLE 4-2: HEMORRHAGIC SHOCK IN INJURED PATIENTS

	CLASS I	CLASS II	CLASS III	CLASS IV
Blood loss (ml)	Up to 750	750-1,500	1,500-2,000	>2,000
Blood loss (%)	Up to 15%	15%-30%	30%-40%	>40%
Pulse rate	<100	>100	>120	>140
Blood pressure	Normal	Normal	Decreased	Decreased
Pulse pressure	Normal or Increased	Decreased	Decreased	Decreased
Respiratory rate	14-20	20-30	30-40	>35
Urine output (ml/hr)	>30	20-30	5-15	Negligible
Central Nervous System	Slightly anxious	Mildly anxious	Anxious; confused	Confused; lethargic
Fluid replacement (3:1 rule)	Crystalloid	Crystalloid	Crystalloid & blood	Crystalloid & blood

Note. Modified with permission from American College of Surgeons' Committee on Trauma, *Advanced Trauma Life Support® for Doctors (ATLS®) Student Manual, 1997; 6th edition,* Chicago: American College of Surgeons, 1997.

TABLE 4-3: CONFOUNDING FACTORS IN TRAUMA PATIENTS' RESPONSE	
Factor	**Caution**
Age	• Elderly trauma patients exhibit limited cardiac reserve and are often unable to generate a tachycardia in response to blood loss. • Consider early invasive monitoring to avoid excessive or inadequate volume restoration.
Athlete	• Blood volume and cardiac output are increased in athletes. Their ability to compensate for hypovolemia may mask significant blood loss.
Pregnancy	• The normal physiologic "hypervolemia" of pregnancy can mask signs of blood loss.
Medication	• Beta-blockers and calcium channel blockers can alter the hemodynamic response to bleeding by blunting tachycardic response.
Pacemaker	• Patients with pacemakers may not generate a tachycardia in response to blood loss.

Blood is lost into the site of the injury. For example, a fracture of the tibia or humerus can lose as much as 750 ml of blood. A fractured femur can lose as much as 1,500 ml of blood. Also be aware that several liters of blood can accumulate in a retroperitoneal hematoma associated with a pelvic fracture. In addition, there is significant edema that occurs in injured soft tissues. The degree of this additional volume loss is related to the magnitude of the soft tissue injury. The tissue injury is associated with systemic inflammatory response and production of cytokines. This leads to increased permeability and fluid shift from the intravascular space into the interstitium, further compromising fluid volume status.

Tip: Note that hypotension in the presence of isolated head injury alone likely points to another injury and requires further assessment and work-up.

INITIAL MANAGEMENT OF SHOCK

The basic principle in the initial management of shock is simply to stop the patient's bleeding and replace volume loss. The diagnosis and treatment of shock occur simultaneously. Following the ABCs helps to keep you organized. Ensure that airway and breathing are established first. Circulation management involves stopping obvious external hemorrhage with direct pressure control. IV fluid resuscitation should ensue, followed by immediate surgery or angiography as necessary. Preventing hypothermia is essential and requires the use of fluid warmers as well as warming blankets. Gastric distention and aspiration is a risk in unconscious patients so nasogastric or orogastric tubes should be inserted early. Foley catheters are required for assessment of urine output monitoring as well as assessment for hematuria. Cardiac monitoring, as well as pulse oximetry monitoring, are essential adjuncts.

Vascular Access

At minimum, two large-bore peripheral IV catheters should be inserted, preferably in the antecubital veins. Size 12- and 14-gauge, short catheters are preferred. The flow rate is directly related to the size of the vessel the catheter is inserted in. Antecubital peripheral IV catheters are preferred over central venous lines, which can cause the added complications of iatrogenic pneumothorax or hemothorax. Within extremis cases, large caliber central venous (femoral, jugular, or subclavian vein) access is recommended. Cordis catheters as large as #9 French can also be used. In children younger than 6 years of age, the placement of an intraosseous needle should be attempted before central line insertion. Intraosseous access with specially designed equipment is also now possible in adults. Use of fluid warmers and rapid infusion devices are also recommended in the face of massive resuscitation. As IV lines are started, blood samples should be drawn for type and crossmatch, additional laboratory analyses, toxicology studies, and the testing of childbearing-age females for pregnancy. Additionally, arterial blood gas analysis is beneficial for all critically ill trauma patients.

Fluid Therapy

In trauma, lactated Ringer's solution is the preferred fluid of choice followed by normal saline solution. Excessive normal saline solution resuscitation can cause hyperchloremic acidosis, especially in the face of decreased renal function. Lactated Ringer's solution brings the added benefit of the lactate changing into bicarbonate when circulating through the liver, which changes it into a buffering solution. This makes it the preferred solution for a trauma patient in shock (American College of Surgeons, 2004a).

Initially 2 L of warmed fluid is given as rapidly as possible. The patient is evaluated for a response. If no improvement is noted, then progression to blood is indicated. A rough guideline to follow is to replace each milliliter of blood loss with 3 ml of IV fluid. This allows for reequilibration of plasma volume that is lost into the interstitial and intracellular spaces. This is known as the "3-for-1 rule." However, it is most important to gauge fluid resuscitation according to the patient's response by continued assessment of vital signs, urine output, and level of consciousness.

Urine Output

Urine output reflects the degree of tissue perfusion and is a useful endpoint in shock resuscitation. Using the weight of the patient best assesses urine output. In the adult, 0.5 ml/kg/hr of urine indicates adequate perfusion. In children, 1.0 ml/kg/hr is

appropriate. For infants, under age 1, 2 ml/kg/hr should be maintained. Urinary output monitoring is one of the prime indicators of resuscitation and should be monitored every 30 min to hourly in the unstable patient.

Acid Base Balance

Early in hypovolemic shock, patients have respiratory alkalosis due to hyperventilation. As shock progresses, the body shifts to anaerobic metabolism, which results in inadequate tissue perfusion, production of lactic acid, and metabolic acidosis. Persistent acidosis as measured by arterial blood gases is an indication of inadequate resuscitation or ongoing blood loss until proven otherwise.

Base Deficit

Base deficit is a useful test to assist guiding trauma resuscitation. Base deficit is defined as the amount of base required titrating 1 L of whole blood to a normal pH at a normal temperature. The base deficit can be determined with each blood gas and is therefore quickly available during resuscitation. The normal range is -2 to +2 mmol/L. It can be ordered every 60 min in an unstable patient and indicates the magnitude of tissue oxygen debt and the adequacy of resuscitation. The more negative the number, the sicker the patient is (see Table 4-4). A progressively negative number means either inadequate fluid replacement or ongoing blood loss. Base deficit of -15 is considered severe and is associated with an increased mortality.

Blood Replacement

The decision to administer blood is based upon the patient's response to initial fluid therapy. Blood is given to restore oxygen carrying capacity of the intravascular volume. The choice of type of blood is dependent on the urgency of the situation.

Emergency Uncrossmatched Blood

For patients in extremis when there is no time to wait for complete blood typing, emergency uncrossmatched blood is warranted. Type O positive blood

TABLE 4-4: BASE DEFICIT IN TRAUMA		
Category	**Base Deficit**	**Mortality**
Normal	+2 to -2	6%
Mild	-3 to -5	11%
Moderate	-6 to -9	23%
Severe	-10 to -15	44%
	-16 to -20	53%
	> -20	70%
(Davis, Parks, Kaups, Gladen, & O'Donnel-Nicol, 1996)		

is given to male trauma patients whereas type O negative blood is reserved for women of childbearing age and children to avoid sensitization and future complications.

Type Specific Blood

Type specific blood has the major ABO and Rh factors identified. Type specific blood is preferred for patients who respond initially to fluids but then deteriorate and require blood quickly. It is generally available within 10 minutes in most blood banks.

Crossmatched Blood

Fully crossmatched blood is preferable whenever possible. However, the complete crossmatch process takes approximately 1 hour in most blood banks. Therefore a blood specimen should be drawn on arrival for all trauma patients.

Hypothermia Prevention

All trauma patients are at risk for developing hypothermia, which is defined as a temperature less than 95° F (35° C). Hypothermia is a frequent pathophysiologic consequence of severe injury and subsequent resuscitation. It is estimated that up to 66% of trauma patients arrive in the emergency department with hypothermia. Hypothermia in the presence of hemorrhage is almost always fatal. Aggressive warming techniques include administration of warmed IV fluids, warmed humidified air, and use of warming blankets (see Table 4-5).

DEFINITIVE CARE

Definitive care for a hemorrhaging trauma patient should be immediate transfer to a facility capable of surgery and/or interventional radiology. A bleeding patient should not remain long in the emergency department but should be promptly moved to the operating room and/or angiography suite for definitive treatment.

SUMMARY

Hypovolemia is the most common cause of shock in trauma patients. Trauma nurses must manage hypovolemia with immediate hemorrhage control and fluid or blood replacement as well as timely preparation for embolization or surgery. The goal of therapy is prompt restoration of organ perfusion with delivery of oxygen. Nurses are pivotal to the trauma team in response to patients in shock.

TABLE 4-5: WARMING STRATEGIES BY DEPARTMENT

Trauma Resuscitation Room	• Turn up the heat in the trauma resuscitation room. • Minimize any draft in the trauma room. Keep the doors shut. • Administer humidified oxygen warmed to 74° F (23° C) via ventilator circuit in an intubated patient. • Remove all wet clothing upon patient arrival. • Minimize body exposure when possible for examination and procedures. • Apply warm blankets. • Promote use of convective air heating devices. • Monitor temperature. • Administer all fluids and blood through a warmer to 76° F (24° C).
Operating Room Interventional Radiology Suite	• Increase room temperature when possible (angiography suite is or routinely kept cold to optimize the machine function). • Cover the patient's head and use heating blankets that permit surgical exposure. • Monitor continuous core temperature. • Ventilate with warmed humidified oxygen at 74° F (23° C). • Administer all fluids and blood through a warmer at 76° F (24° C). • Assess for the onset of hypothermia, acidosis, and coagulopathy. • Anticipate temporary closure of the abdomen using alternative techniques.
Critical Care Unit	• Increase patient room temperature. • Keep door of room closed. • Continue head covering and convective warming blanket use. • Coordinate and minimize exposure for all procedures. • Monitor core temperature continuously. • Administer all fluids and blood through a warmer at 76° F (24° C). • Ventilate with warmed humidified oxygen at 74° F (23° C).

EXAM QUESTIONS

CHAPTER 4

Questions 23-32

23. Which of the following best characterizes a diagnosis of shock?

    a. Evidence of inadequate organ perfusion

    b. Systolic blood pressure below 90 mm Hg

    c. Pulse pressure less than 20 mm Hg

    d. Alkalosis on blood gas

24. The most common cause of inadequate perfusion in trauma patients is

    a. inadequate cardiac contractility.

    b. decreased circulating blood volume.

    c. inadequate vasomotor tone.

    d. increased cellular permeability.

25. Compensatory mechanisms in shock include

    a. increased peripheral vasoconstriction.

    b. decreased sympathetic tone.

    c. decreased heart rate.

    d. increased blood flow to the gut.

26. The first drop in systolic blood pressure occurs in which class of hemorrhagic shock?

    a. Class I

    b. Class II

    c. Class III

    d. Class IV

27. Vasoconstriction is seen in

    a. early septic shock.

    b. anaphylactic shock.

    c. cardiogenic shock.

    d. neurogenic shock.

28. Which of the following indicates shock that may have a cause other than hypovolemia?

    a. Distended neck veins

    b. Hypotension

    c. Decreased pulse pressure

    d. Decreased skin temperature

29. Confounding variables in patient response to hemorrhage include

    a. tachycardia in elderly patients.

    b. the normal hypertension of pregnancy.

    c. increased cardiac output in athletes.

    d. tachycardia from beta-blocker use.

30. A 16-year-old male is brought into the emergency department after crashing his car into a cement wall at high speed. He is unconscious and in obvious shock with a blood pressure of 60/40 and a pulse rate of 150. He has no open wounds or obvious fractures. The cause of his shock is most likely caused by

    a. epidural hematoma.

    b. subdural hematoma.

    c. transected spinal cord.

    d. hemorrhage into the chest or abdomen.

31. A 20-year-old male arrives at a trauma center with a gun shot wound to the abdomen. He is in Class IV shock with a tachycardia of 156 and blood pressure of 78/40. He is immediately prepped and leaves for the operating room. Which blood administration is appropriate?

    a. Emergency uncrossmatched Type O positive

    b. Emergency uncrossmatched Type O negative

    c. Type specific blood

    d. Crossmatched blood

32. Which of the following nursing interventions is the most aggressive warming treatment for the hypothermic trauma patient?

    a. Gastric lavage with room temperature saline

    b. Increased room temperature

    c. Cloth blankets

    d. Warmed ventilator humidified air and IV fluids

CHAPTER 5

HEAD INJURY

CHAPTER OBJECTIVE

Upon completion of this chapter, the reader will be able to describe the principles of proper management of head injuries.

LEARNING OBJECTIVES

Upon completion of this chapter, the reader should be able to

1. identify the major areas of the brain and their functions.

2. recognize the signs and symptoms of increased intracranial pressure (ICP).

3. differentiate the signs and symptoms and classification of head injuries.

4. recognize the importance of the Glasgow Coma Scale (GCS) in the assessment of a patient with a head injury.

5. indicate appropriate interventions for head-injured patients.

INTRODUCTION

Traumatic brain injury (TBI) is the leading cause of trauma deaths. Nearly 75% of all victims of fatal motor vehicle crashes (MVCs) demonstrate brain injury on autopsy (Moore et al., 2004). Approximately 500,000 cases of brain injury occur in the United States annually. The cost in terms of death and disability, along with medical, rehabilitative, loss of productivity, and psychosocial impact is tremendous. The paradox of the emergency medical services (EMS) system is that because of improved training and technology, more traumatic head and spine injury victims are saved, but there are also now more severely disabled people who require costly extensive rehabilitation and lifelong maintenance and care.

Most of the victims of traumatic head injuries are between ages 15 and 24 who have been involved in MVCs (Ferrera et al., 2001). To further complicate the injuries, often the patient has alcohol or drugs, legal or otherwise, in the vehicle. Although the mandatory use of seat belts and campaigns against drunk driving have decreased traffic fatalities by an estimated 25%, the incidence of penetrating injury to the brain and spinal cord is increasing. Gunshot wounds play a major part in penetrating trauma. Other leading causes of head trauma are recreational injuries and falls.

The faster a head injury is identified, assessed, and interventions begun, the better the patient's potential for survival with minimized disabilities.

ANATOMY AND PHYSIOLOGY

The severity of head injuries is high because there is little support or protection for the head.

Understanding the basic anatomy and physiology of the head and brain is essential for the most appropriate assessment and initial interventions for head injuries (see Figure 5-1).

FIGURE 5-1: ANATOMY OF THE HEAD

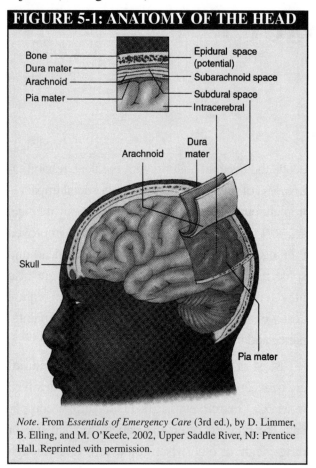

Bone
Dura mater
Arachnoid
Pia mater

Epidural space (potential)
Subarachnoid space
Subdural space
Intracerebral

Arachnoid

Dura mater

Skull

Pia mater

Note. From *Essentials of Emergency Care* (3rd ed.), by D. Limmer, B. Elling, and M. O'Keefe, 2002, Upper Saddle River, NJ: Prentice Hall. Reprinted with permission.

Scalp

The scalp is the thickest layer of body covering but thins with age and balding. It provides spongy protection for the skull. There are five layers: skin, subcutaneous tissue, galea aponeurotica, ligaments, and periosteum. The tissue is highly vascular, and it does not take a large laceration to cause a lot of bleeding. Uncontrolled bleeding can result in significant blood loss. Direct pressure can usually control the bleeding.

Skull

The skull, or cranium, functions as a container to hold and protect the brain. It is composed of the frontal, parietal, temporal, and occipital bones. Cranial bones join with the facial bones to form the cranial vault, which is a rigid cavity. An opening called the foramen magnum allows the spinal cord to pass through.

Other important areas are the depressions in the interior base of the skull called the anterior, middle, and posterior fossa. The anterior fossa contains the frontal lobe, which coordinates voluntary movements and controls judgment, affect, and personality. The parietal, temporal, and occipital lobes are in the middle fossa. The parietal lobe controls sensory interpretation; the temporal lobe controls hearing, behavior, emotions, and dominant-hemisphere speech; and the occipital lobe is responsible for vision. The brain stem and cerebellum are in the posterior fossa.

The temporal area is especially thin, making it extremely vulnerable. The base of the skull is rough and has irregularities that can bruise and lacerate the brain when the head is jarred suddenly or in rapid deceleration. The solid structure of the adult skull makes it unable to tolerate expansion of the brain or increase in volume without serious problems.

Meninges

Inside the skull there are three highly vascular layers of membranes, the meninges that surround and protect the brain and the spinal cord. The outer layer is the dura and is the thickest and toughest of the three layers. The meningeal arteries are located in a space between the skull and the dura called the epidural space.

Lying under the dura is a weblike transparent serous membrane called the arachnoid.

The third layer, the pia, is attached to the brain and the arachnoid in some areas.

Brain

Made up of billions of nerve cells, the adult brain weighs about 3 pounds and occupies approximately 80% of the intracranial space. Brain tissue is the most energy-consuming tissue in the body and receives about 20% of the body's oxygen supply

(McQuillan, Truter von Rueden, Hartsock, Flynn, & Whalen, 2002). Brain cells cannot go more than 4 to 6 minutes without oxygen before irreversible damage occurs, unless they are in a hypothermic state and the metabolism is drastically slowed.

The brain has three distinct parts: the cerebrum, brain stem, and cerebellum. The cerebrum is divided into two hemispheres, the left and right. Each hemisphere has lobes named for their corresponding part of the skull. They control specific intellectual, sensory, and motor functions.

The brain stem joins the spinal cord, serving as a key reflex and relay center for the central nervous system. Consciousness, breathing, heart rate, and "vegetative functions" are controlled here. The cerebellum surrounds the brain stem in the posterior fossa and coordinates activities below the level of consciousness, such as posture and equilibrium.

Inside the brain are a series of four interconnected cavities called ventricles. Cerebrospinal fluid (CSF) is produced here. It bathes the outer surface of the brain and acts as a shock absorber between the brain and the skull, along with serving as a blood-brain barrier against harmful substances.

Cranial Nerves

Twelve pairs of cranial nerves originate in the brain stem, with each separate nerve having a name and a Roman numeral identifier. These nerves have unconscious control over sensory, motor, or both activities. Functions and areas they affect are important to recognize because they are instrumental in the accurate assessment of damage from a head injury because they are indicators of brain stem activity and neurologic function.

The most important cranial nerve for assessment of a head injury is the third, or oculomotor, nerve that controls pupillary constriction. In a patient with an altered level of consciousness, a nonreactive or sluggish pupil indicates damage or pressure to the third nerve. This nerve is frequently injured in head trauma patients.

Pediatric Differences

A child's head is disproportionately large for the body size, and the neck is comparatively weak. The cranial bones are thinner, and the brain tissue is thinner, softer, and more fragile than an adult. Consequently, there is a greater chance that cerebral edema will develop in a child than in an adult. However, pediatric patients often have a better recovery from a trauma brain injury.

CONDITIONS OF HEAD INJURIES

Increased Intracranial Pressure

Unconsciousness stems from pathology in either the cerebral cortex or the reticular activating system in the brain stem. Because the brain is in an enclosed area, as pressure increases in the head, it causes the cerebral blood flow and thus available oxygen to decrease, which in turn, causes the level of consciousness to diminish. This is called the Monroe-Kellie doctrine (see Figure 5-2).

If there is a swelling in one part of the brain, it compresses another area because the skull cannot expand. If the whole brain swells, or there is a rapidly growing hematoma, it takes up the limited intracranial space, compressing the blood vessels and decreasing blood flow.

The pressure in the arteries of the skull is considerably higher than the increased intracranial pressure (ICP). When the ICP increases enough to equal the pressure in the skull's arteries, these vessels are squeezed, further restricting blood flow. The body responds to the decrease in blood flow and the resulting drop in blood pressure by stimulating the sympathetic nervous system. This causes even more vasoconstriction, which further increases the blood pressure. Additionally, the pulse slows because of the pressure on the vagus (X cranial) nerve. Respiratory response alters the breathing pattern.

FIGURE 5-2: MONROE-KELLIE DOCTRINE: INTRACRANIAL COMPENSATION FOR EXPANDING MASS

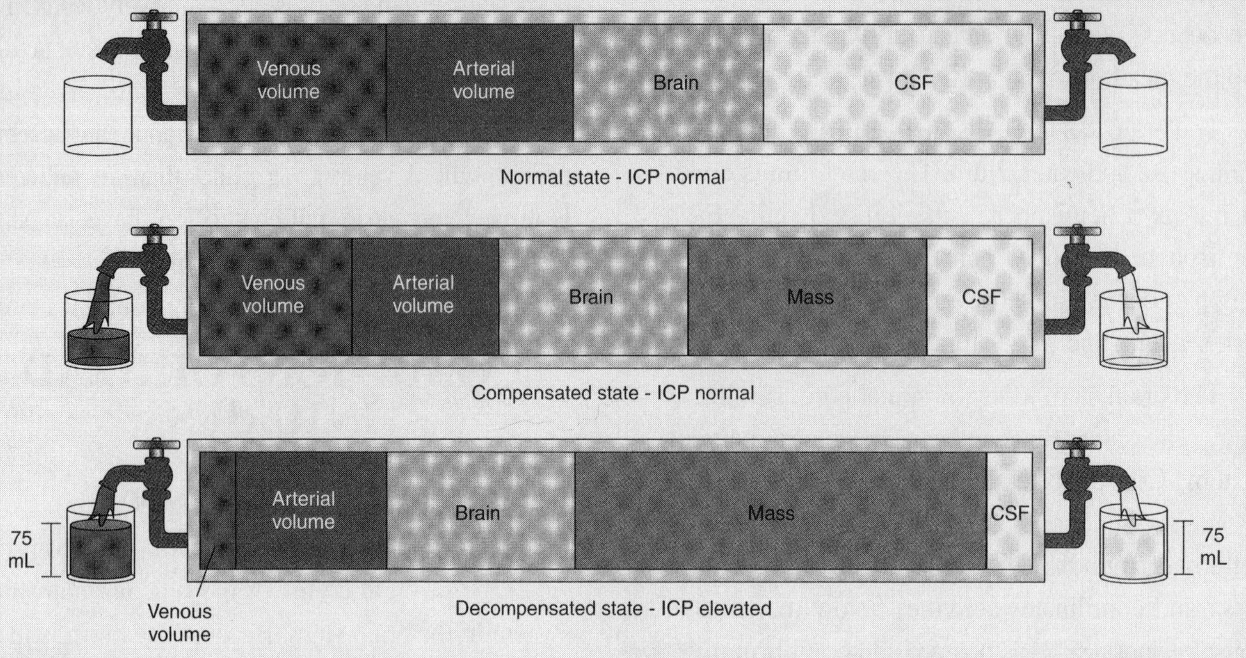

Note. From *PHTLS Basic and Advanced Prehospital Trauma Life Support*, (5th ed.), 2003, St. Louis, MO: Mosby. Reprinted with permission from Elsevier.

Tip:

- The triad of rising blood pressure, slowing pulse rate, and changing respiratory pattern is an extremely late sign of increasing ICP.

- Earlier signs and symptoms of increasing ICP may include decreased level of consciousness, pupil changes, weakness, nausea, vomiting, headache, seizures, and an abnormal respiratory pattern.

The increasing ICP causes a decreased level of consciousness, deficits in vital functions, and can lead to brain death from inadequate cerebral perfusion. If the response to the increased ICP becomes exhausted, the brain begins to shift and can herniate through the tentorium above the cerebellum, causing death.

SPECIFIC HEAD INJURIES

Trauma is physical injury to the body from an external force, at times severe enough to endanger a person's limbs or life. The mechanism of injury may be either blunt or penetrating.

Most brain injuries are caused by blunt trauma to the head, especially in MVCs. When a vehicle hits an object it stops, but the occupant continues forward, crashing into the interior of the vehicle. As the person hits the interior of the vehicle and stops, the brain continues to move forward, striking the skull. As the brain hits the skull during the deceleration injury, it absorbs energy and rebounds to the opposite side of the skull. The first contact of the brain with the skull is called the coup and the rebound collision with the skull is called the contrecoup.

Penetrating injuries create wounds through the skull. Usually a fracture occurs, and the projectile may drive bone fragments along with a foreign body into the brain, causing damage along the way. Intracranial bleeding and structural damage result. When impalement is the source of the penetrating injury, the object lodged in the head should be left in place and stabilized while the patient is being evaluated. Removal could worsen the effects from the injury.

CLASSIFICATIONS OF HEAD INJURY

Head injuries are classified in several ways. They can be classified by mechanism, severity, and morphology (see Table 5-1).

Mechanism of Injury

Head injury can be broadly as blunt or penetrating. Blunt injury is associated with MVCs, falls, and blunt assaults. Penetrating injury usually results from gunshot and stab wounds.

Severity of Injury

The Glasgow Coma Scale (GCS) score is used as an objective clinical measurement of the severity of brain injury (see Table 5-2). The GCS is used to measure level of consciousness and should be repeated at least hourly to determine whether the patient's neurologic status is improving or deteriorating. The total score results from a cumulative score of the best eye response, best verbal response, and best motor response. The lowest possible score is 3 and the highest is 15. A GCS score of 14 to 15 indicates mild head injury and a GCS score of 9 to 13 is categorized as moderate, while a GCS score below 8 is generally accepted as severe brain injury or coma.

TABLE 5-1: CLASSIFICATION OF HEAD INJURIES		
Mechanism	Blunt	MVCs, falls, assaults
	Penetrating	Gunshot wounds
Severity	Mild Moderate Severe	Glasgow Coma Scale (GCS) score 14-15 GCS score 9-13 GCS score 3-8
Morphology	Scalp	Scalp lacerations

	Skull Fractures
	
	     Vault
	
	     Basilar
		
		Linear versus stellate
		Depressed versus nondepressed
		Open versus closed
		
		With and without cerobrospinal fluid leak
		With and without VII nerve palsy

	Intracranial Lesions Focal	 Contusions Epidural Subdural
	Diffuse	Concussion Multiple contusions Hypoxic ischemic injury

TABLE 5-2: GLASGOW COMA SCALE	
BEST EYE RESPONSE	
Spontaneously	4
To voice	3
To pain	2
Remain closed	1
BEST VERBAL RESPONSE	
Oriented	5
Confused	4
Inappropriate words	3
Make sounds	2
No response	1
BEST MOTOR RESPONSE	
Obeys commands	6
Localizes stimulus	5
Withdraws from stimulus	4
Abnormal flexion	3
Abnormal extension	2
No response	1
Total Score	3 (minimum) 15 (maximum)

Sample GCS Scoring

A 33-year-old female pedestrian presents to the trauma center after being struck by a car at 50 mph. There is a large bleeding head wound noted on the right parietal region. She does not respond to verbal stimuli. Pressure is applied to her nail beds. See the following patient responses and fill in the GCS score to the left of the response.

Then calculate her GCS and grade the severity of brain injury.

Score	Action
____	She opens her eyes.
____	She moans and grunts.
____	She pulls her hand away.
____	Total GCS

Answers: Eye = 2, Verbal = 2, Motor = 4.
Total GCS is 8, indicating severe brain injury.

Focal Injuries

Focal injuries have a specific area of involvement and diffuse injuries involve the entire brain.

Scalp Laceration

As stated earlier, the scalp is highly vascular and bleeds profusely, even with a small laceration. While a laceration may cause a considerable amount of blood loss, it is not likely to be life threatening. Direct pressure will usually initially control the bleeding, followed with wound repair.

Skull Fracture

A skull fracture may or may not be immediately obvious. The clinical picture directly correlates to the type of fracture, area, and structures damaged. If there is no occurrence of associated brain injury, CSF leak, hematoma, or subsequent infection, skull fractures are not of serious consequence to the patient.

Skull fractures may be seen in the cranial vault or skull base (see Figure 5-3). They may be linear or stellate, and may be open or closed. Do not underestimate the significance of a skull fracture. It takes considerable force to fracture the skull.

A linear fracture is caused by blunt trauma, is nondisplaced, and usually has minimal neurological deficit. Eighty percent of skull fractures are linear. Supportive care is generally all the patient needs.

FIGURE 5-3: TYPES OF SKULL FRACTURES

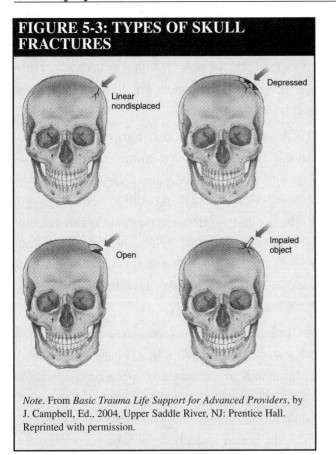

Note. From *Basic Trauma Life Support for Advanced Providers*, by J. Campbell, Ed., 2004, Upper Saddle River, NJ: Prentice Hall. Reprinted with permission.

If the impact has enough force, the fracture may be depressed, with bony fragments being driven into the brain. The depressed fracture will require surgical intervention if bone fragments become lodged in the brain tissue. When the damage to the skull causes an open wound or laceration, surgical repair is urgent to control bleeding and pressure in the brain and manage the risk of infection.

Basilar fractures may result from an extension of a linear fracture to the floor of the skull. Most commonly, these fractures occur through the floor of the anterior cranial fossa from craniofacial injuries, and may cause enough damage for the CSF to leak through either the nose (rhinorrhea) or ears (ottorhea). Carotid artery and cranial nerve injuries are also frequently seen with basilar fractures, in particular, the facial nerve paralysis (cranial nerve VII).

Basilar fractures may not be visualized on an x-ray or computed tomography (CT) scan; so clinical findings may have to be relied on for the diagnosis.

Bleeding can cause dramatic distinguishing changes in the appearance of the patient. When blood leaks into the periorbital tissue, it causes what is known as "raccoon's eyes." Another characteristic is "Battle's sign," ecchymosis behind the ear seen 12 to 24 hours after the initial injury. Other clinical signs of fracture are CSF leaks from the nose or ears. Neurologic changes with a basilar fracture range from slight alteration in mental status to agitation or severe combativeness, depending on the injury to underlying brain cells.

Contusion

When the brain hits against the cranium it becomes bruised, particularly in acceleration-deceleration trauma. Usually these are coup and contrecoup injuries. Depending upon the size and location of the contusion, neurological deficit may or may not be evident. Increased ICP will result from a large contusion. Symptoms include alteration of consciousness, nausea, vomiting, visual and speech difficulties, and weakness.

Epidural Hematoma

Epidural hematomas result from a direct strike to the head, causing a bleed between the skull and dura mater (see Figure 5-4). Epidural hematomas are most commonly located in the temporal region where the middle meningeal artery is torn and a hematoma can form rapidly.

FIGURE 5-4: EPIDURAL HEMATOMA

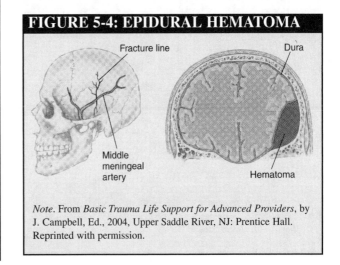

Note. From *Basic Trauma Life Support for Advanced Providers*, by J. Campbell, Ed., 2004, Upper Saddle River, NJ: Prentice Hall. Reprinted with permission.

Signs of a rapidly growing hematoma and increasing ICP are loss of consciousness (LOC) followed by a lucid period (usually a hallmark of an epidural bleed), followed by another LOC period; developing hemiparesis; and a dilated and fixed pupil on the side of impact. The triad of increasing blood pressure, slowing pulse rate, and changes in respiratory patterns are ominous signs of elevated ICP. Signs and symptoms of an epidural hematoma depend on the rate of blood accumulation. Clinical manifestations are usually seen within 6 hours of injury (McQuillen et al., 2002). An epidural hematoma creating a significant mass effect requires immediate operation for evacuation of the clot and ligation of bleeding vessels. Once the LOC decreases and there is presence of a unilaterally dilating pupil, the patient must immediatly be operated on.

Subdural Hematoma

Occurring more frequently than other intracranial injuries, subdural hematomas have the highest morbidity and mortality of all intracranial hematomas. They are usually the result of venous bleeding between the dura and the brain and frequently are associated with brain tissue damage (see Figure 5-5).

Subdural hematomas are classified as acute, subacute, and chronic. Acute hematomas are often caused by high-velocity impact injuries and have a

grave prognosis because of the underlying brain injury. Even with immediate surgical intervention, more than 50% of patients will not survive the damage. Clinically, the patient has LOC; hemiparesis; and fixed, dilated pupils.

A subacute hematoma, also caused by high-impact trauma, develops more slowly, from 48 hours to 2 weeks. The patient experiences a progressive decline in LOC proportionate to the growth of the hematoma. Because the brain is able to compensate for the gradual collection of blood, the neurologic functions deteriorate slowly. These patients have a better prognosis than those with acute hematomas.

In the chronic hematoma, week to months after what seemed like a minor head injury, blood slowly accumulates in the subdural space or between the layers of the dura. Since the causative injury occured previous to the symptoms becoming evident, the actual incident may have been forgotten. Older adults frequently have this type of injury. Their brain decreases in size due to atrophy, thus allowing more blood to collect in the increased intracranial space before symptoms become noticeable. Although it takes more time to recognize the chronic subdural hematoma, the mortality rate is almost as high as that of the acute subdural hematomas.

DIFFUSE INJURIES

Diffuse brain injuries range from mild concussions where the head CT scan is usually normal to severe hypoxic ischemic injuries. With concussion, the patient may have a brief LOC and may suffer from amnesia.

Severe diffuse injury usually occurs from an hypoxic insult to the brain due to prolonged shock or loss of airway after the trauma. The CT scan may initially appear to be normal or may appear diffusely swollen with loss of the normal white-gray interface. Less commonly there may be multiple

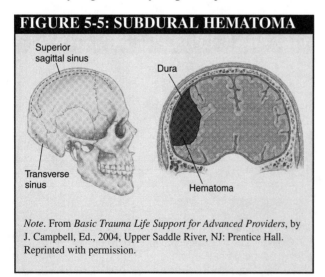

FIGURE 5-5: SUBDURAL HEMATOMA

Superior sagittal sinus

Dura

Transverse sinus

Hematoma

Note. From *Basic Trauma Life Support for Advanced Providers*, by J. Campbell, Ed., 2004, Upper Saddle River, NJ: Prentice Hall. Reprinted with permission.

punctuate hemorrhages throughout the cerebral hemispheres. Severe hypoxic ischemic, injuries formerly known as DAI (diffuse axonal injury), generally have a poor outcome. Diffuse injuries usually are not visible lesions, as with focal lesions, but are injuries to several microscopic axons of the brain.

Concussion

A concussion occurs from a direct blow or acceleration-deceleration injury where there is temporary LOC and associated memory deficiency without underlying brain damage. Injury is not severe. There may be temporary amnesia. Headache, nausea, vomiting, and visual disturbances are also likely to be experienced. It is important to determine any incidence and length of LOC, neurologic status, and memory deficits.

Postconcussion syndrome will exhibit headache, memory loss, and diminished activities of daily living. The symptoms can last for as long as a year after the injury.

PATIENT ASSESSMENT

Immediately immobilize the patient's head and neck and secure the airway. Support breathing with 100% oxygen with a nonrebreather mask or bag-valve mask device as indicated. All patients with head injuries should be continuously monitored to determine if their neurologic status is constant, improves, or deteriorates. Change may occur on a minute-to-minute basis.

Loss of Consciousness

Assessment of LOC involves determining the highest level of response with the least stimulus. Even the subtlest change from the initial assessment provides early indication of deterioration or improvement in the patient's condition. Repeated GCS assessment and documentation provides immediate recognition of deterioration.

Pupils

Normally, pupils constrict with direct-light examination. Observation of unilaterally fixed and dilated pupils may indicate oculomotor nerve compression from increased ICP and herniation. A mildly dilated pupil with sluggish response may also be an early sign of herniation. Bilateral fixed and pinpoint pupils may indicate pontine lesion or adverse effects of drugs (opiates) (see Figure 5-6).

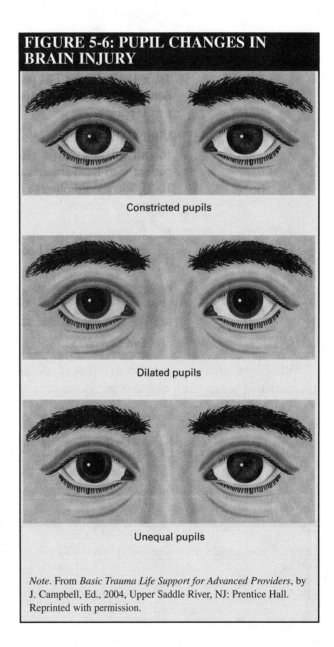

FIGURE 5-6: PUPIL CHANGES IN BRAIN INJURY

Constricted pupils

Dilated pupils

Unequal pupils

Note. From *Basic Trauma Life Support for Advanced Providers*, by J. Campbell, Ed., 2004, Upper Saddle River, NJ: Prentice Hall. Reprinted with permission.

Posturing

Posturing and unequal motor responses indicate brain injury (see Figure 5-7). Decorticate (flexion) and decerebrate (extension) posturing are ominous signs of brain injury, however decerebrate is worse and may signify cerebral herniation. Flaccid paralysis usually indicates spinal cord injury.

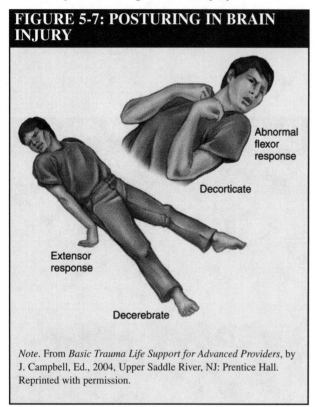

FIGURE 5-7: POSTURING IN BRAIN INJURY

Abnormal flexor response

Decorticate

Extensor response

Decerebrate

Note. From *Basic Trauma Life Support for Advanced Providers*, by J. Campbell, Ed., 2004, Upper Saddle River, NJ: Prentice Hall. Reprinted with permission.

Vital Sign Changes

Vital signs change in relation to different conditions, such as trauma, shock, and ICP (see Table 5-3).

Respiratory Rate

Patients with a GCS of below 8 require immediate intubation. If the neurological deterioration is not identified immediately, then respiratory changes will be noted. Respirations may slow, become rapid, uneven, and noisy, or the patient may develop respiratory embarrassment or deteriorate into cardiopulmonary arrest.

Blood Pressure

Hypotension in the presence of isolated head injury should make one suspect there is a missed injury elsewhere. Hypotension is not associated with head injuries alone and its cause should be aggressively pursued. Blood pressure elevation in head injuries can be indicative of the increasing ICP. Increased blood pressure, slowing pulse rate, and changing respiratory pattern are all ominous signs of ICP.

Heart Rate

As previously discussed, the development of bradycardia may reflect increased ICP. Bradycardia with hypertension can be due to a rapidly expanding hematoma. The pulse rate is an important factor to be evaluated with other assessment data to determine if it is related to the head injury.

It cannot be over emphasized that continuous assessment and recording of results are essential in the management of the patient's care.

TABLE 5-3: COMPARISON OF VITAL SIGNS IN SHOCK AND HEAD INJURY		
	SHOCK	HEAD INJURY WITH INCREASED ICP
Level of consciousness	Decreased	Decreased
Respiration	Increased	Varies but often decreased
Pulse	Increased	Decreased
Blood pressure	Decreased	Increased
Pulse pressure	Narrows	Widens

Note. From *Basic Trauma Life Support for Advanced Providers*, by J. Campbell, Ed., 2004, Upper Saddle River, NJ: Prentice Hall. Reprinted with permission.

Monitoring Increased Intracranial Pressure

Catheters are inserted into the brain and connected to a monitor for ICP continuous monitoring. Normal ICP is approximately 10 mm Hg. Pressures greater than 20 mm Hg are generally considered abnormal. ICP monitoring is indicated for patients with a GCS score below 8 after resuscitation and an abnormal admission CT scan. ICP should be continuously monitored for the first 3 to 5 days post severe head injury. Hourly documentation of ICP at minimum is required.

TREATMENT STRATEGIES

Avoid Secondary Insult: Hypotension and Hypoxia

Brain injury is adversely affected by secondary insults, such as hypotension and hypoxia. Oxygenation and IV hydration are essential in preventing secondary injury. Patients with severe head injury and hypotension on admission have more than double the mortality as compared with patients without hypotension. The addition of hypoxia to hypotension substantially increases the mortality even more. Therefore it is imperative that cardiopulmonary stabilization occurs quickly in severely brain-injured patients.

Preventing Aspiration

The head-injured patient is likely to vomit. Care must be taken to prevent aspiration. Turn the backboard or logroll the patient to the side. Keep suction equipment available for use at any time. Do not insert tubes into the nose if there are suspected midface fractures. Orogastric tube placement is often indicated.

Oxygenation

Provide high flow oxygenation and monitor oxygenation with a pulse oximeter. Protect the airway if LOC deteriorates. Intubation is indicated for all head injured patients with a GCS below 8.

Control Blood Loss

Identify and control all sources of blood loss. Because scalp vessels bleed profusely, it may be difficult to visualize the site. Probing through the laceration or wound to observe depth or search for foreign bodies should be avoided. The vessels are easily compressed with gentle, continuous direct pressure. Avoid direct pressure over obvious deformity, palpable bony defects, or instability. Instead, apply gentle pressure around the wound, taking care to exert pressure only on stable bone. Excessive blood loss from scalp injuries is particularly a problem in children with head injury.

Maintain Cerebral Perfusion

Adequate cerebral perfusion pressure (CPP) is a function of the difference between the mean arterial blood pressure (MAP) and ICP. [*CPP = MAP - ICP*] As ICP increases, CPP decreases, leading to cerebral ischemia. Therefore, it is important to keep the blood pressure up and avoid hypotension. This measure offsets the effect of increasing ICP. Strategies to address CPP are discussed next.

Fluid Resuscitation to Optimize Mean Arterial Blood Pressure

As with any trauma patient, IV fluids and blood administration ensure adequate perfusion of all organs. Lactated Ringer's and/or normal saline solution are the preferred solutions in head-injured patients. Hypotonic solutions such as dextrose 5% in water (D_5W) should be avoided because they reduce the osmolarity of intravascular volume, which encourages fluid leakage out of the intravascular space, thereby exacerbating cerebral edema. Continuous invasive blood pressure monitoring is essential along with close observation of urine output and base deficit to monitor fluid resuscitation. The use of hypertonic saline is still under investigation but appears promising (Moore et al., 2004).

Strategies to Control Increased Intracranial Pressure

- Elevate the head of the bed to 30 degrees for increased ICP after spine injury has been ruled out.

- Consider sedation and paralysis of the intubated patient to avoid any straining or movement that will cause increased ICP.

- Hyperventilation should be avoided and is only reserved for brief periods for acute severe neurologic deterioration. Maintain a Pco_2 between 35-40 mm Hg.

- Mannitol, an osmotic diuretic, can be used to reduce elevated ICP. Typical dosing range is 0.25 to 1 g/kg of body weight of a 20% solution as a bolus. (McQuillen et al., 2002). Bolus dose administration is preferred rather then continuous infusion. It is also preferable to administer mannitol through a central line because extravasation can cause skin sloughing. Monitor urine output and hemodynamic status carefully when using large doses of mannitol in hypotensive patients because of its osmotic diuretic effects.

- Barbiturate coma may be used on occasion when increased ICP is refractory to other measures.

- Insertion of a ventriculostomy catheter allows for drainage of excess CSF.

Seizure Control

Anticonvulsants should be considered for head-injured patients, especially those with early onset seizures, intracranial hematoma, and depressed skull fracture. Posttraumatic epilepsy is known to occur in up to 5% of all head injuries. Careful assessment of airway, ventilation, and oxygenation are important after seizure.

DEFINITIVE CARE

Anticipate the need for prompt CT scans and immediate need for surgery. Consider early transfer to a trauma center with neurosurgery capabilities.

DISCHARGE CARE

Send head injury discharge instructions home with all mild head-injured patients discharged from the emergency department to a responsible family member.

BRAIN DEATH

The diagnosis of brain death means that there is no chance for brain function recovery. The clinical criteria for the declaration of brain death include (McQuillen et al., 2002):

1. Known cause of death

2. Irreversibility

3. Nonreactive pupils

4. Body temperature > 63° F (17° C)

5. Absence of spontaneous movements in response to external stimuli

6. No reflex activity except that elicited by spinal cord

7. Apnea in the presence of hypercapnia ($Paco_2$ > 60 mm Hg)

SUMMARY

Injuries to the head are the leading cause of traumatic deaths and significant disabilities. MVCs involving people between ages 15 and 24 are the predominant cause of these injuries.

Knowledge of the anatomy and physiology of the head along with the dynamics of head injuries is fundamental to identifying types of head injuries and conducting effective initial and secondary assessments. All patients with potential or obvious head trauma need to be continuously monitored because of the potential for a rapid change in status. The faster the head injury is identified, assessed, and interventions are initiated, the better the patient's potential for minimized injuries and survival.

EXAM QUESTIONS

CHAPTER 5

Questions 33-39

33. Head injuries are severe because

    a. the scalp provides only a thin protection.

    b. the cranial nerves are easily damaged.

    c. there is little support or protection for the head.

    d. the brain is so large.

34. Late signs of increasing ICP can be best characterized by

    a. increased respiration.

    b. increased pulse rate.

    c. increased systolic blood pressure.

    d. narrowed pulse pressure.

35. Focal head injuries

    a. are more severe than diffuse injuries.

    b. involve a specific area of the brain.

    c. are rarely fatal.

    d. usually penetrate the skull.

36. An unhelmeted 20-year-old female is thrown from a horse and arrives at the emergency department (ED). She responds to verbal stimuli with eye opening and confused speech. She has purposeful movement and can follow commands. What is her GCS?

    a. 9

    b. 13

    c. 14

    d. 15

37. The most important initial step in the treatment of a head injury is

    a. control scalp hemorrhage.

    b. obtain c-spine film.

    c. determine GCS.

    d. secure the airway.

38. Nursing interventions aimed at preventing secondary brain injury is

    a. administering of an osmotic diuretic.

    b. raising the head of the bed.

    c. ensuring adequate IV fluid hydration and oxygenation.

    d. reducing metabolic requirement of the brain.

39. A construction worker arrives at the ED after being hit in the head with a large steel pipe at a construction site. His GCS is 6, he has a palpable depressed skull fracture, and has gurgling respirations. There is vomitus on his face and clothing. The most appropriate initial nursing intervention is to

    a. suction the airway.

    b. administer oxygen via bag-valve mask.

    c. administer oxygen via nonrebreather mask.

    d. prepare for immediate orotracheal intubation.

CHAPTER 6

MAXILLOFACIAL AND NECK TRAUMA

CHAPTER OBJECTIVE

Upon completion of this chapter, the reader will be able to recognize the causes and management of maxillofacial and neck trauma.

LEARNING OBJECTIVES

Upon completion of this chapter, the reader should be able to

1. identify the anatomy and related functions of the face and neck.

2. recognize causes and symptoms of maxillofacial and neck trauma.

3. recognize common traumatic injuries of the eye.

4. select appropriate interventions to treat maxillofacial, neck, and ocular trauma.

INTRODUCTION

Maxillofacial and neck trauma are frequently seen injuries in the emergency department. Motor vehicle crashes (MVCs) are the most common cause, but physical assaults, personal altercations, and handguns are increasing contributors to facial and neck trauma. Falls are also a frequent cause of these injuries in older adults and children.

Eye injuries are frightening because of the fear of resulting vision defects or loss. Injuries may be obvious, as with penetrating trauma, or difficult to detect, particularly in an unresponsive patient who has multiple injuries. True traumatic emergencies of the eye are quite rare, even more rare to be life threatening.

Facial trauma includes the facial bones, neurovascular structures, skin, subcutaneous tissue, muscles, glands, and the upper airway. It takes significant force to fracture the midface or maxilla, and as a result, multisystem injuries usually accompany these types of fractures. When there are multiple injuries, maxillofacial trauma is a complicating factor.

Assessing even a severe facial injury does not take priority over recognition and treatment of life-threatening injuries. As in every injury, rapidly checking airway, cervical spine stabilization, breathing and circulation come first. Maxillofacial and neck trauma may appear severe, but usually is not critical unless the airway is compromised. Patients with trauma to the neck can be at high risk because the airway, carotid vessels, jugular vessels, and cervical spine are all contained in this compact area. Specific head and spinal injuries are discussed in other chapters.

ANATOMY AND PHYSIOLOGY

Eye Structures

The eye, shaped like a globe, is approximately 1 inch (2.5 cm) in diameter, about 80% of which sits in a bony structure of the skull called the orbit (see Figure 6-1). Six oculomotor muscles move the eye and are innervated by cranial nerves IV and VI.

The eyelids protect the eyes. Their inner surfaces are moistened with tears produced by the lacrimal (tear) glands. Every time the eye blinks, the lids cover the exposed surface to clean away dirt and other irritants and bathe it with tears. The tears are then drained through the lacrimal duct, which leads to the nasal cavity.

The white of the eye is the sclera. It is a semi-rigid capsule made up of fibrous tissue surrounding the globe that helps to maintain its shape and contain the fluids within the eye.

The colored portion of the external eye, the iris, is a contractible membrane suspended between the lens and the cornea. The iris is often used as an identifier of people by its color, and it surrounds an adjustable opening called the pupil.

A clear portion of the sclera, the cornea, lies over the iris and pupil as protection. It helps to keep the fluids in the eye and plays an important part in focusing light.

Covering the sclera and the cornea and lining the surfaces of the eyelids is the conjunctiva. It lubricates the tissues that make contact with the air. When the tiny vessels in the conjunctiva become swollen with blood, the eyes look pink or "bloodshot."

The interior of the eye is divided into an anterior and posterior chamber. The anterior chamber is located between the cornea and the lens. It is filled with a clear, watery fluid, the aqueous humor, which circulates through the anterior and posterior chambers. If the aqueous fluid leaks and is lost through a penetrating injury, it will replace itself with proper treatment.

The colorless lens is enclosed in a capsule and is suspended behind the iris and the pupil. As light rays pass through the cornea and the aqueous

FIGURE 6-1: ANATOMY OF THE EYE

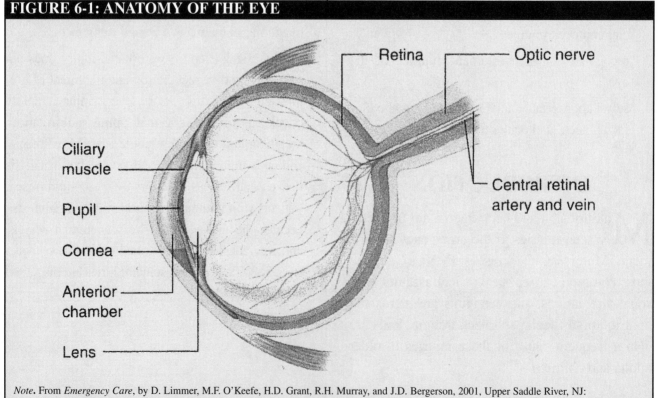

Note. From *Emergency Care*, by D. Limmer, M.F. O'Keefe, H.D. Grant, R.H. Murray, and J.D. Bergerson, 2001, Upper Saddle River, NJ: Brady Prentice Hall. Reprinted with permission.

humor, they bend, which is the beginning of the focusing process. The light continues through the transparent lens. Muscle action changes the shape of the lens to make it thicker or thinner, which controls how the light reaches the retina.

The lens is the dividing structure between the anterior and posterior chambers. The entire posterior cavity is located behind the lens and is filled with a transparent jelly-like substance called the vitreous humor. The vitreous humor is important in maintaining the shape and length of the globe. It exerts a degree of pressure on the lens so that the lens is able to function properly. Vitreous humor cannot be replaced, and it cannot regenerate itself. If the vitreous humor is lost, the eye is lost.

The retina is the innermost lining of the eyeball and lines the entire interior of the eye. It extends from where the optic nerve (cranial nerve II) enters at the back of the globe to the margin of the pupil.

The retina is light sensitive where the rays focus to receive the image formed by the lens. The cells of the retina convert light into electrical impulses that are conducted through the optic nerve to the vision center (occipital lobe) at the back of the head.

Facial Structures

The skull functions as a rigid container. There are two specific areas, the cranial vault and the 14 facial bones. The structures of the face, jaw, and neck form part of the upper airway.

The main facial bones are the frontal, nasal bone, maxilla, zygoma, and mandible (see Figure 6-2). All of the facial bones touch the maxillae.

The **frontal** bone or forehead joins to the frontal process of the maxilla, the nasal bone, and laterally to the zygoma.

The **orbital complex** is a bony pyramid-shaped cavity in the skull that contains and protects the eyes. It is comprised of the frontal bone, zygoma, and maxilla. Posteriorly is the optic foramen, a groove for the optic nerve and ophthalmic artery at the orbit's apex.

The **maxilla**, also called the midface, are two bones that meet in the midline of the face. They

FIGURE 6-2: THE HUMAN SKULL

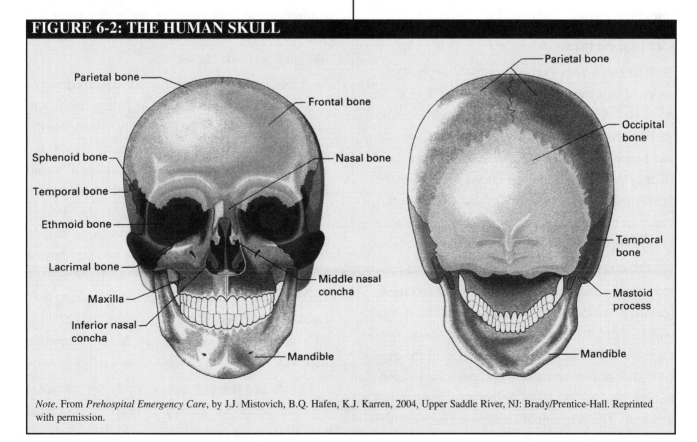

Note. From *Prehospital Emergency Care*, by J.J. Mistovich, B.Q. Hafen, K.J. Karren, 2004, Upper Saddle River, NJ: Brady/Prentice-Hall. Reprinted with permission.

form the skeletal base of most of the upper face. Included are most of the orbital floor, sides of the nasal cavity, the upper jaw, and the roof of the mouth, which also houses the upper teeth.

The **sinus cavities** in the midline of the face lighten the weight of the bony structure and act as resonating chambers. They develop from the nasal cavities, communicate with them, and are filled with air. Their specific function is not known.

The **nose** is made up of a pair of bones that form the bridge, is mostly made of cartilage, and protrudes from the face, making it vulnerable to injury. The nasal cavity is divided by the septum.

The **zygoma** forms the cheek and the lateral wall and floor of the orbital cavity. The zygoma articulates with the maxilla, frontal bone, and zygomatic process of the temporal bone to form the zygomatic arch.

The **mandible** is horseshoe shaped, lies horizontally, and is the only movable bone in the face. It is the strongest bone and anchors the lower teeth. The mandible articulates with the temporal bone to form the temporomandibular joint.

Cranial Nerves

The **facial nerve** (cranial nerve VII) gives sensory and motor innervation to the side of the face. It originates in the brain stem and then subdivides into six branches, leading to the scalp, forehead, eyelids, and facial muscles for expression, cheeks, and jaw. Injuries to the facial nerve produce a paralysis to the facial muscles; a possible loss of taste, and a disturbance in the secretion of the lacrimal and salivary glands, depending on the part of the nerve involved.

Other nerves that can be affected by facial trauma are the **oculomotor** (cranial nerve III), **trochlear** (cranial nerve IV), and **abducens** (cranial nerve VI), which innervate the ocular muscles. Injuries can produce blurred vision; diplopia; deviation of the eyeball; impaired ocular movements; ptosis, or inability to open the eye; and affect the ability of the pupil to constrict. The **trigeminal** (cranial nerve V) is the largest of the cranial nerves. Trauma can cause paralysis of the muscles used to chew; inability to clench the jaw; loss of ability to feel light tactile, thermal and painful sensations to the face; and loss of the corneal and sneezing reflexes.

Upper Airway

The hyoid bone is U-shaped and attached to the base of the tongue. It does not touch any other bone. Because of its attachment to the tongue, it is likely to obstruct the airway.

The passages from the nose and mouth meet at the **pharynx** or throat. The pharynx begins at the base of the skull and opens into the esophagus and the larynx. It is muscular and is divided into the nasopharynx behind the nasal cavities (containing the adenoids and openings to the eustachian tubes) the oropharynx extending from the uvula to the epiglottis (containing the palatine tonsils), and the laryngopharynx that extends from the epiglottis to the opening of the larynx. Here, constrictor muscles send food and liquid into the esophagus. The gag reflex and swallowing is controlled by the **glossopharyngeal nerve** (cranial nerve IX). The pharynx may become obstructed with food, liquids, or foreign bodies such as teeth.

From the pharynx, the **larynx** extends down to the upper end of the trachea. A leaf-shaped structure just behind the root of the tongue and attached to the thyroid cartilage is the **epiglottis**. It covers the entrance to the larynx during swallowing, allowing food to go down the esophagus and keeping food, liquid, and foreign objects out of the airway. Although the larynx assists in speech, it mainly functions as an air passage opening into the **trachea** or the "windpipe." Vocal cords project into the larynx from the trachea, and when they spasm, they cause choking. The larynx can close, allowing for air buildup in the lungs, which can be forcefully expelled, known as a cough.

Extending from the upper airway, the trachea is the main passage to convey air from the upper airway in and out of the lungs. It is supported by C-shaped cartilage connected by a tough membrane, through which an opening can be made for artificial ventilation during upper airway obstruction or a crushing injury of the neck.

Neck Anatomy

Major Vessels

Carotid arteries run alongside the trachea on either side of the neck, arise from the aorta, and are the principal blood supply to the head and neck. Both the right and left carotids divide to form the internal and external carotid arteries. Chemoreceptors in the arteries respond to changes in blood chemistry, such as hypoxia, and cause reflex increases in pulse rate, blood pressure, and respiratory rate. If the blood supply to the head is interrupted, brain ischemia will occur. When a carotid pulse can be palpated, the systolic blood pressure is approximated to be at least 60 mm Hg.

Jugular veins

The external jugular vein receives blood from the exterior of the cranium and the deep parts of the face. It lies superficially to the sternocleidomastoid muscle as it descends the neck to join the subclavian vein. The internal jugular vein receives blood from the brain and superficial parts of the face and neck. It runs alongside the internal carotid artery and joins the subclavian vein to form the innominate vein.

Laceration or a tear of the carotid arteries or jugular veins can rapidly lead to exsanguination. Air can also be drawn into the venous vessels and form a fatal air embolus.

MECHANISM OF INJURY

Blunt maxillofacial or neck trauma can range from an uncomplicated nasal fracture to a major head injury or the collapse of the upper airway. Frequently, rapid deceleration and forceful impact with a hard surface are the mechanism for trauma to the face or neck. MVCs, sports accidents,

falls, or impact from assault are the most frequently seen sources of these injuries.

Blunt trauma to the eye may be caused by MVCs, assault, a fall, or other direct blow to the eye. Injuries range from minor corneal abrasions or contusions to retinal detachment or the loss of an eye. Most often, the injury is to the orbit rather than the eyeball. Projectiles, such as a knife or a missile, cause most penetrating injuries to the eyeball. Injury may affect the surface of the eye or the globe. Damage includes laceration, impalement, or puncture, any of which threaten vision or the eye itself. Often these injuries occur due to the lack of protective eyewear. Burns also cause ocular trauma and are an immediate threat to vision. Burns can be chemical, heat-related, or radiation.

OCULAR INJURIES AND INTERVENTIONS

Foreign Body

Foreign bodies to the eye most often are small particles, such as pieces of dirt, dust, or metal shavings. The particle may be seen on the surface of the cornea with the naked eye, or it may require a magnifier, such as a slit lamp, to be identified. Organic foreign bodies are more likely to cause infection, and metallic objects will leave a rust ring unless removed within 12 hours. The patient will have pain (especially when the eyelid is opened and closed), copious tearing, and sensitivity to light. The pain is similar to that of a corneal abrasion. The foreign body must be located and removed, which may require local anesthesia for effective treatment.

Corneal Abrasion

A scratch or scrape to the cornea is likely to be caused by a foreign object and is a common occurrence. Contact lens scratches are frequent. Normally, the cornea appears smooth, clear, wet, and moist. An abrasion is rarely visible to the naked eye without fluorescein staining. Injury can abrade or denude the epithelium and expose the superficial corneal nerves, which causes pain, tearing, and eyelid spasms. Antibiotic ointments are applied, and the eye should be patched for 24 hours. Patching prevents eyelid movement and further irritation to the eye.

Hyphema

Blunt trauma causing a bleed into the anterior chamber of the eye is referred to as hyphema. The size of a hyphema ranges from small to complete involvement of the anterior chamber. "Eightball hyphema" is total involvement that has started to clot. The sclera may appear bloody. Blood in the anterior chamber may be seen in persons with light-colored eyes, but in those with dark eyes, it can be extremely difficult to see. Clinical management is directed toward reducing the risk of rebleeding. The injured eye should be shielded and, if possible, the patient should be positioned sitting upright or with the head of the bed elevated. Cycloplegic or mydriatic drops may be ordered to reduce or prevent a ciliary spasm.

Retinal Detachment

Retinal detachment is not truly a detachment where the entire retina separates from the choroid (a vascular layer between the sclera and the retina). Instead, the pigment layer of the retina remains attached to the choroid and the rest of the retina detaches from it. The detachment may have a tear. When a tear occurs, the vitreous seeps between the layers. Additionally, the loss of blood and oxygen supply makes the retina unable to see light and disrupts impulses to the optic nerve. A detachment can occur from various medical causes, a hole or break in the inner sensory layer, or can be precipitated by trauma. Treatment includes possible laser repair or scleral buckling for a torn retina, bed rest, and patching both eyes.

Chemical Burn Injury

The primary signs and symptoms of a corrosive chemical burn to the eye include severe burning pain, swelling of the lids, and rapid onset of visual impairment. The delicate tissues of the eye are easily damaged permanently. The emergency treatment for chemical burns is flushing the eye with sterile water or normal saline solution. However, if nothing else is available, tap water should be used. Copious irrigation takes priority even over assessment. The eye may have to be held open so that it can be adequately flushed. Irrigation should be gentle and not forceful to prevent increased pain or further damage to the tissue. Irrigation should be continued for as long as it takes to get the conjunctival pH to a normal range of 7.4 to 7.6. Cycloplegic agents are generally ordered to reduce pain from a ciliary spasm. Cover the eye with a moist dressing.

MAXILLOFACIAL AND NECK INJURY

Soft-Tissue Trauma

Contusions are a frequent result of blunt trauma that does not alter the integrity of the skin. Pain, swelling, and discoloration is the result of extravasation of blood into the damaged tissue. Around the eyes, a contusion may indicate an orbital fracture.

Animal or human bites are highly contaminated because of the bacteria and debris in the mouth. Extensive or gaping wounds present infection and cosmetic problems, along with the possibility of foreign bodies entering the wound.

Road rash and friction injuries have the potential problems of tattooing or epidermal staining. Gunpowder can also cause permanent discoloration and cosmetic disfigurement, along with burns to the epithelial and collagen layers while penetrating the skin. Glass fragments are often embedded in the skin after the head has gone through a windshield.

Soft-tissue injury from air bags can cause minor abrasions to the face, neck, and upper chest. Occasionally, air bags cause scleral or corneal injury and lacerations to the eyebrows and eyelids. Ear injuries and deafness can also occur.

Lacerations are open cuts caused by a shearing force through the layers of the skin. They range from simple to deep cuts and are associated with crush injuries and fractures. For cosmetic reasons, lacerations of the face require special attention.

Lacerations of the lips require the skills of a plastic surgeon so the vermilion borders can be perfectly matched and "step-off" deformities of the lip do not develop.

Ear injuries are classified as hematomas, lacerations, and avulsions. Hematomas that are not drained can result in a "cauliflower ear," which is a scar deformity. Cartilage may be lacerated along with the skin. Avulsion injuries are more involved than simple lacerations and require skin preservation so grafting from other body areas is not required.

Facial nerve injury can be overlooked if the patient is unconscious or has multiple facial bandages. Facial paralysis from blunt trauma, rather than laceration, has a good chance of recovery if the damage is not extensive.

An avulsion is the tearing of a flap of skin from the body surface. It may be completely removed or stay partially attached to the body. The injury usually causes a lot of bleeding, requiring immediate direct pressure.

Major Vessel Injury

Penetrating trauma to the neck is a serious emergency. Laceration of a great vessel can cause hemorrhaging; air can get sucked in and cause an embolus. It is difficult to stop this type of hemorrhaging because of the pressure in the vessels.

The carotid arteries are the major neck arteries and suppliers of blood to the head. They supply the blood for perfusion and oxygenation of the brain. Bright red, spurting blood in a pulsating flow from an open neck wound indicates a carotid artery may be damaged, which is an extreme emergency.

Dark red venous blood streaming from an open neck wound is an acute emergency because of the potential blood volume loss and possibility of air entering the venous system, producing an air embolus. Direct pressure with immediate surgical repair is required.

Neck Injuries

Penetrating trauma of the neck is classified as injury to Zone I, II, or III (see Figure 6-3). The importance of these zones is related to 1) identification of structures potentially injured, 2) decision for deciding on selective surgical management or observation with diagnostic testing, and 3) potential to control bleeding.

Any patient with neck trauma who presents with hemodynamic instability, exsanguinating hemorrhage, an expanding hematoma, air-bubbling wound, subcutaneous emphysema, or stridor requires immediate surgical exploration. Caution is required when treating a penetrating injury to the neck. There often are no findings suggestive of injury to a vital structure. Many of these injuries will remain silent until causing complications later. Specifically injuries to the larynx, trachea, esophagus, cervical spine, and carotid arteries must be ruled out. Therefore it is necessary to perform diagnostic tests to rule them out within the first 8 to 12 hours of admission. The most common diagnostic tests used are laryngoscopy, tracheoscopy, bronchoscopy, esophagoscopy, and arteriography. A surgical exploration is performed only when and if a specific injury is found.

Fractures

Nasal Fracture

Because the nose is the most prominent facial feature and offers the least resistance, it is the most common facial fracture. The mechanism is usually blunt trauma. If left untreated, deformity can result,

FIGURE 6-3: ZONES OF THE NECK

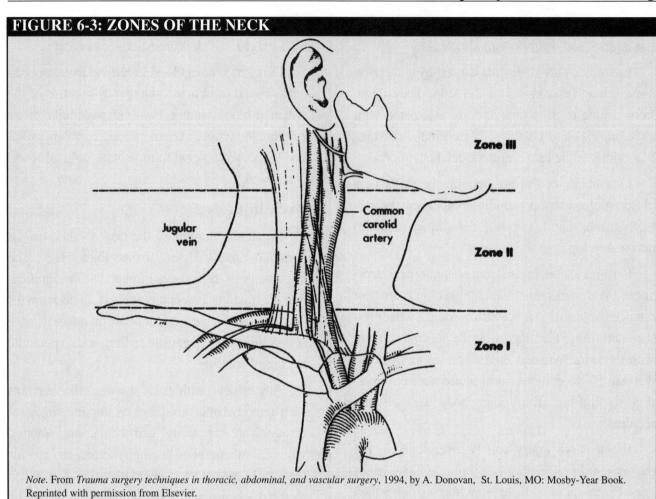

Zone III

Common carotid artery

Zone II

Jugular vein

Zone I

Note. From *Trauma surgery techniques in thoracic, abdominal, and vascular surgery,* 1994, by A. Donovan, St. Louis, MO: Mosby-Year Book. Reprinted with permission from Elsevier.

along with airway obstruction. When the overlying skin is broken, the fracture is open.

A septal hematoma presents as a bluish, bulging mass. Emergency aspiration of the hematoma is required to prevent airway obstruction, septal necrosis, and a permanent deformity. A blow from the side of the nose can cause lateral displacement. Bleeding from nasal trauma can be profuse, being intranasal as well as in the pharynx. If a fracture involves the nasal mucosa of the lacrimal system, blowing the nose can cause intracranial air or subcutaneous emphysema that may subsequently become localized infection or meningitis.

Mandibular Fracture

The second most frequent type of facial fracture is mandibular. A forceful blow from MVCs, sports, or altercations are the usual mechanism of injury. Loss of bony support, in a mandibular fracture can be

life threatening if it displaces posteriorly and blocks the airway. Malocclusion is the most prominent symptom, but symptoms vary with the location of the fracture. The face may be asymmetric with swelling and ecchymosis. Sublingual hematomas can compromise the airway. There may also be tears in the external canal of the ear or the tympanic membrane.

Maxillary Fracture

It takes great force to cause a midface fracture, and usually there are other fractures involved. There are three different types of maxillary fractures (see Figure 6-4).

LeFort I is a lower-third fracture that is horizontal, where the body of the maxilla is separated from the base of the skull above the palate but below the zygomatic process attachment. Separation may be unilateral or bilateral, and the maxilla may be displaced. The hard palate and the upper teeth are loose.

FIGURE 6-4: LEFORT FRACTURE TYPES

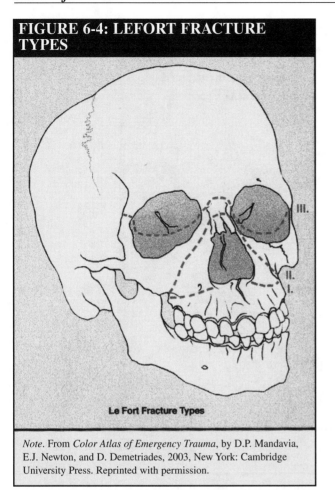

Le Fort Fracture Types

Note. From *Color Atlas of Emergency Trauma*, by D.P. Mandavia, E.J. Newton, and D. Demetriades, 2003, New York: Cambridge University Press. Reprinted with permission.

LeFort II is a middle-third fracture including the central maxilla, nasal area, and ethmoid bones. The nose, lips, and eyes are usually edematous; subconjunctival hemorrhage and epistaxis frequently occurs. Cerebrospinal fluid rhinorrhea suggests skull fracture.

LeFort III is an orbital complex fracture causing total cranial facial separation. The nose and dental arch move without frontal bone involvement accompanied by massive edema, ecchymosis, epistaxis, and malocclusion. Ocular injuries are secondary to the swelling. Airway obstruction, likely from hemorrhage and cervical spine fracture, should always be considered.

Zygoma Fracture

Zygomatic fractures occur in two patterns: zygomatic arch and tripod (see Figure 6-5). Fracture of the cheeks most often occurs from blunt trauma to the front or side of the face. If there is also a fracture of the orbital floor, the situation may become critical.

FIGURE 6-5: ZYGOMA FRACTURE

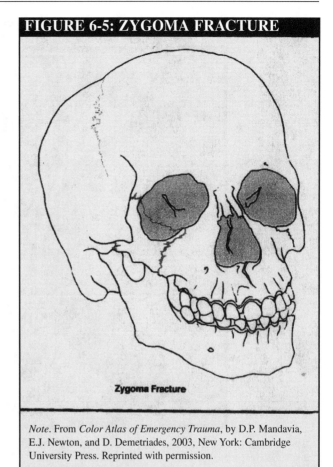

Zygoma Fracture

Note. From *Color Atlas of Emergency Trauma*, by D.P. Mandavia, E.J. Newton, and D. Demetriades, 2003, New York: Cambridge University Press. Reprinted with permission.

Orbital Blowout Fracture

Orbital blowout and zygoma fractures can occur separately, but are often found together. The orbital blowout is caused by a direct blow to the eye causing the globe to "blowout" or fracture one or more bones of the orbital wall (see Figure 6-6). The weakest part of the orbit is the floor.

Increased pressure can cause the orbit's contents to prolapse into the maxillary sinus, causing entrapment of the inferior rectus muscle, inferior oblique muscle, infraorbital nerve, orbital fat, and connective tissue. The globe may also become entrapped.

When the globe is perforated, blowing the nose or manipulating the eyes can cause intraorbital air. If there is subcutaneous orbital emphysema, a fracture of the sinus arch should be suspected. Nose blowing, coughing, sneezing, vomiting, and straining can force air from the sinuses through the fracture into the orbital space. If there is bulging of the eye and limitation of motion, ocular involvement is

FIGURE 6-6: BLOWOUT FRACTURE OF THE ORBITAL FLOOR

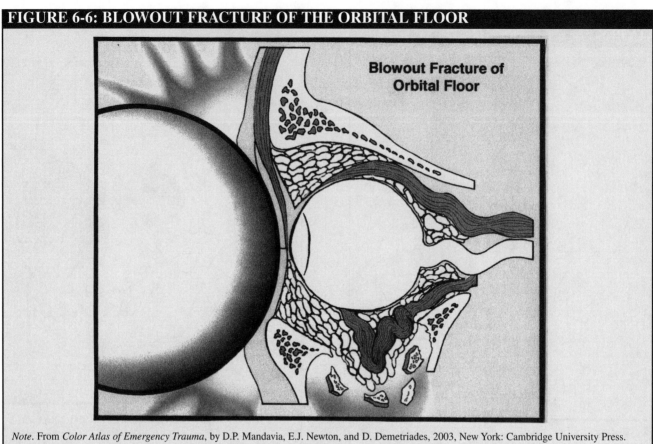

Blowout Fracture of Orbital Floor

Note. From *Color Atlas of Emergency Trauma*, by D.P. Mandavia, E.J. Newton, and D. Demetriades, 2003, New York: Cambridge University Press. Reprinted with permission.

a consideration. Double vision, pupil asymmetry, sunken appearance of the globe, anesthesia of the cheek and upper lip, or drooping of the lid are all indicators of a blowout fracture.

ASSESSMENT

Primary Assessment

As with any head or neck injury, particularly if the patient is unconscious, the primary assessment assumes there is a cervical fracture. Stabilization of the neck, a clear airway, and adequate oxygenation are the first priorities.

There are many causes for airway obstruction in cases of head and neck injury. When the facial structures are damaged or the tongue is left without support, occlusion of the airway is likely. Foreign objects, such as avulsed teeth or dentures, can also obstruct the airway. A fracture of the nasoorbital complex compromises the airway due to hemor-

rhage. Altered mental status or injury may decrease the gag reflex, leaving the airway unprotected.

Identify serious injuries that threaten the patient's life or limbs and stop any uncontrolled bleeding.

Secondary Assessment

Once the neck is stabilized, the airway open, the patient adequately ventilated, and hemorrhage controlled, the secondary assessment should be conducted.

Maxillofacial injuries seldom are life threatening unless there is a compromised airway. However, there are likely to be other associated fractures.

INTERVENTIONS

*   Stabilize the neck with cervical collar placement.
*   Monitor the airway for patency. Midfacial fractures can cause airway obstruction. If there is airway compromise, perform immediate jaw thrust and prepare to intubate.

- Elevate the head of the bed to reduce swelling, bleeding, congestion, and to promote drainage, once the spine has been cleared.

- Suction as needed. If the patient is alert, promote self-suction with a tonsil tip catheter.

- Apply ice packs and direct nasal pressure to control swelling and bleeding from the nose.

- Avoid insertion of a nasogastric tube or nasal airway in a patient with a suspected midfacial or basilar skull fracture. Place an orogastric tube instead.

- Apply sterile dressing to control facial or scalp bleeding with direct pressure, except where there is an obvious fracture, a ruptured or penetrated eyeball, leaking cerebrospinal fluid, or exposed brain tissue.

- Secure impaled objects to avoid movement.

- Save loose or dislodged teeth. Put them in moist gauze or a container with saline or milk, and label them with the date, time, and patient's name. They may possibly be reimplanted if performed quickly.

- When applying pressure to bleeding from the neck, be sure to restrict blood loss but not to occlude the airway. Keep in mind the potential of air being sucked into the jugular vein and the formation of an air embolus. Keep the wound covered with a wet, sterile dressing.

- Never shave the eyebrows of a patient with facial trauma. They do not grow back and are needed as landmarks for repair.

- Remove contact lenses.

- Instruct the patient not to bend forward, cough, or perform a Valsalva maneuver as these actions may raise intraocular pressure.

- Instill prescribed topical anesthetic drops for pain control and to facilitate eye examination except in open globe injuries.

- Instill normal saline solution drops or artificial tears to keep the corneas moist, as indicated.

- Cover the eyelids with a sterile, moist saline dressing to prevent corneal drying and ulceration.

- Lightly patch or shield both eyes to reduce movement and photophobia in patients with retinal injuries.

SUMMARY

Maxillofacial and neck injuries are the most frequent types of injuries seen in the emergency department. Maxillofacial injury can be dramatic in appearance, often because of hemorrhaging or disfigurement from fractures. Although usually not life threatening, the involvement of facial bones, neurovascular structures, skin and subcutaneous tissue, and glands can be complicating factors in the management of patients with multiple injuries.

EXAM QUESTIONS

CHAPTER 6

Questions 40-43

40. An indication of a mandibular fracture is

    a. Battle's sign.

    b. malocclusion.

    c. carotid artery involvement.

    d. LeFort's syndrome.

41. A motorcycle driver sustained a clothesline injury to his neck at high speed. You would expect to find which of the following

    a. subcutaneous emphysema.

    b. Kerh's sign.

    c. Cushing's triad.

    d. Battle's sign.

42. Which of the following are characteristics of an orbital blowout fracture?

    a. Bulging appearance of the globe.

    b. Pupil symmetry is common.

    c. Results from direct blow to the eye.

    d. The muscles of the eye are not involved.

43. A patient is brought into the emergency department with maxillofacial trauma after being accidentally shot in the face. Your initial assessment reveals a large cheek wound; there is blood in his airway, his radial pulse is weak and rapid. Which is your first priority?

    a. Suction the airway.

    b. Apply oxygen with a nonrebreather mask.

    c. Insert a nasopharyngeal airway.

    d. Ventilate with a bag-valve mask.

CHAPTER 7

THORACIC TRAUMA

CHAPTER OBJECTIVE

Upon completion of this chapter, the reader will be able to indicate the major nursing strategies for managing thoracic trauma.

LEARNING OBJECTIVES

Upon completion of this chapter, the reader should be able to

1. identify physical assessment techniques that help to identify thoracic injuries.

2. recognize the signs and symptoms of common chest injuries.

3. choose appropriate interventions to manage chest injuries.

INTRODUCTION

The thoracic cavity, or chest, contains organs, structures, and vessels of the pulmonary, cardiovascular, and gastrointestinal systems. These systems, structures, and vessels are vital to life, and because of that, any damage to the chest is potentially serious. Because the body is unable to store oxygen, a chest injury interfering with normal respiration or the functioning of any of these three systems is emergent.

Thoracic trauma is a significant cause of mortality. Chest trauma accounts for 20% of all trauma deaths and is the second most common cause of all trauma deaths after head injury (Ferrera et al., 2001). Many trauma patients with thoracic injuries die after reaching the hospital. Appropriate management immediately upon arrival to the emergency department can prevent unnecessary deaths. Only about 10% of blunt chest trauma require thoracotomy while up to 30% of penetrating chest trauma require immediate operation (American College of Surgeons, 2004b).

Today, about 85% of the trauma cases can be managed nonoperatively with analgesia, good pulmonary toilet (coughing and deep breathing), chest roentgenography, selective endotracheal intubation, and tube thoracostomy (Ferrera et al., 2001).

ANATOMY AND PHYSIOLOGY

The thorax, or chest, which extends from the top of the sternum to the diaphragm, is one of two major body cavities; the other is the abdominal cavity. Boundaries are the 12 pairs of ribs that articulate with the thoracic spine posteriorly and with the sternum anteriorly. The clavicles overlie the upper boundaries in front and join with the scapulae in the muscle tissue of the back. The superior border of the thorax is continuous with the neck. The lower boundary is the diaphragm, which separates the thoracic and abdominal cavities. Patients with penetrating injuries below the nipple line anteriorly or inferior to the scapula posteriorly, most likely also have abdominal damage. Figure 7-1 depicts the anatomy of the thoracic cavity.

FIGURE 7-1: THE THORACIC CAVITY

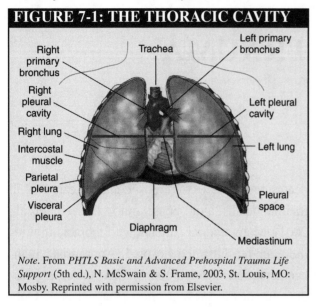

Right primary bronchus
Trachea
Left primary bronchus
Right pleural cavity
Left pleural cavity
Right lung
Left lung
Intercostal muscle
Parietal pleura
Visceral pleura
Pleural space
Diaphragm
Mediastinum

Note. From *PHTLS Basic and Advanced Prehospital Trauma Life Support* (5th ed.), N. McSwain & S. Frame, 2003, St. Louis, MO: Mosby. Reprinted with permission from Elsevier.

Within the thorax are structures, organs, and vessels of the pulmonary, cardiovascular, and gastrointestinal systems. The pleural space contains the pulmonary organs, and the mediastinal space contains the cardiovascular and gastrointestinal structures.

Important structures in the thorax are the ribs, sternum, lungs, pleurae, intercostal and accessory muscles, diaphragm, trachea, esophagus, heart, and great vessels. Twelve pairs of ribs form the rib cage, which is meant to function as a chest protector. The centrally located sternum provides additional protection but can function as a weapon to the heart and lungs if it is fractured. Essential to life by providing oxygen to the body and removing carbon dioxide, the lungs fill most of the chest and are covered by the visceral pleura. The trachea funnels air in and out of the lungs, subdividing into bronchi and bronchioles. The esophagus, which lies behind the trachea, is a tube for transporting food into the gastrointestinal system. Under the sternum, slightly to the left, lies the heart with important vessels entering and leaving it and the lungs.

PULMONARY SYSTEM

One lung occupies each half of the chest cavity, or the hemothorax. Between the lungs is a space, the mediastinum, where the heart, great arteries and veins, many nerves, esophagus, trachea, and major bronchi are located.

The lungs hang freely within the chest cavity. Because they are not made up of muscle, they have no ability to expand or contract on their own.

There is a mechanism to ensure the lungs follow the motion of the chest wall, expanding and contracting with it. A thin membrane, the parietal pleura, lines the inner surface of the chest cavity. The same kind of serous membrane, the visceral pleura, also covers the surface of each lung. Between the visceral pleural surface of the lungs and the parietal pleural surface of the chest wall is the so-called pleural space. In reality, this space is a "potential" space, because the visceral pleura and the parietal pleura actually lie against each other, sealed tightly with a thin film of fluid. An analogy would be two panes of glass stuck together by a thin coating of water. When the chest wall expands, the lung is pulled with it and made to expand by the pulling force of the two pleural layers.

Under normal conditions, no real space exists between the pleural layers, because the fluid causes them to adhere to each other. However, if traumatized, the potential space can hold 3,000 ml or more in an adult. For instance, if the chest wall is lacerated, blood can separate the pleural surfaces and fill the space. A hole in the chest wall or a torn lung can cause air to enter the pleural space. In either case, the pleurae are no longer sealed together, and the means for them to expand the lungs is lost. If enough blood or air collects, the lungs can be compressed to the degree that they cannot expand at all during inspiration. At this point, there will not be enough oxygen to maintain life.

The mechanics of breathing are three-dimensional. As discussed, the lungs do not contain muscle tissue and cannot expand or contract on their own. The intercostal and accessory muscles of the thorax along with the movement of the diaphragm cause expansion in three directions; out, up, and down. The attachment of the lungs to the pleural surfaces causes them to follow the expanding motion of the chest wall, permitting air to enter the airways and the alveoli.

Although the diaphragm is skeletal or voluntary muscle (in that one can control taking a deep breath, coughing, or controlling breathing patterns at will), it also performs an automatic function. Breathing occurs while asleep or awake. Conscious variations in breathing, such as holding one's breath, cannot continue indefinitely. When the balance of oxygen and carbon dioxide is disturbed enough, automatic regulation of respiration takes over.

NEGATIVE PRESSURE

The chest can be thought of as a bell jar in which the lungs are suspended. The only natural opening into the chest is the trachea through which air moves in and out of the lungs. Ordinarily, the pressure in the chest cavity is slightly less than the atmospheric pressure. When the chest wall muscles and diaphragm contract during inspiration, the ribs expand and the diaphragm drops, so the thorax space enlarges, and the volume the chest can hold is increased.

The increased space causes the intrathoracic pressure to drop further and develop a slight vacuum. The result is that the higher outside pressure drives air through the trachea, filling the lungs. As the air moves in, the inside pressure begins to equal the pressure outside, and when it does, the air stops moving. The principle is that any gas will move from a higher-pressure area to a lower-pressure area until the pressure in each area is equal. In the case of ventilation, when the pressures are equal, inspiration stops. At this point, expiration begins. The intercostal muscles and diaphragm relax, the chest

contracts and becomes smaller, the pressure inside becomes higher than the pressure outside, and the air is expelled.

The key point is that the trachea is the only natural opening for air to enter the chest cavity. If there is another opening from an injury, the air cannot get to the interior of the lung through the trachea, because air or blood enters the pleural space through the injury, breaks the pleural seal, compresses the lung, and effectively stops normal chest expansion.

CARDIOVASCULAR SYSTEM

The cardiovascular system is the engine that keeps the body running, delivering oxygen and nutrients and disposing of cellular waste and carbon dioxide. Working as a closed circuit, the heart pumps the blood and makes the system go. The system is not simple. It is a complex arrangement of systemic circulation (the transport of blood throughout the body to exchange oxygen, nutrients, and waste products) and pulmonary circulation (the transport of blood through the lungs to exchange oxygen and carbon dioxide).

The heart, large vessels, trachea, esophagus, thymus, and lymph nodes are situated in the mediastinum, a cavity between the lungs. The heart is positioned slightly on the left half of the chest, with the right ventricle lying beneath the sternum. The pericardium, a tough, layered sac that cannot expand, surrounds and protects the heart similar to the pleurae around the lungs. It is made up of an inner layer, the visceral pericardium and an outer layer, the parietal pericardium. As with the pleural space, the pericardial cavity is a potential space between the two-pericardial layers that is filled with a small amount of serous fluid. The fluid serves to prevent friction during heartbeat. The parietal pericardium attaches to the sternum, great vessels, and diaphragm in order to hold the heart in place.

The right heart is a low-pressure system, receiving deoxygenated blood and pumping it to the lungs for oxygenation. Oxygenated blood returns to the left heart, a high-pressure system, to be pumped through the systemic circulation. Cardiac output and function depend on contractility, heart rate, preload, and afterload. Preload is the volume reached after diastolic filling of the ventricles. Afterload is the resistance the heart pumps against to push the blood out.

There are three anatomical portions of the aorta: the ascending aorta, aortic arch, and the descending aorta. Just distal to the arch, the aorta is quite immobile and at risk for disruption. The vast majority of aortic injuries are caused by acceleration/deceleration forces to the descending aorta.

MECHANISM OF INJURY

The chest can be injured by blunt trauma, penetrating objects, and compression mechanisms. The extent of injury depends upon the force, direction, duration, and physical area where the traumatic energy impacts.

Blunt Trauma

A majority of the chest injuries are caused by blunt trauma, in particular, by rapid deceleration, most often in car crashes. Energy rebounds through the thorax and may crush soft tissues against the spine, rupturing organs. Blunt trauma with force sufficient to fracture the rib cage, sternum, or costal cartilage can result in heart or lung contusion. Rapid vertical deceleration can shear the aorta and great vessels from the heart.

Penetrating Object

Any sharp object having enough force will cause a penetrating injury. Penetration injuries can result in localized or widespread damage as a result of bullets, knives, shards of metal or glass, and a variety of other objects that can pierce the chest.

Penetrating injuries can lacerate, impale, puncture, or rupture an organ, structure, or vessel. Stab wounds may not appear damaging but can have significant morbidity and mortality from deep penetration into the chest and its contents. Bullet wounds usually have a clear point of entry and exit, with the line of damage being obvious, but the bullet may ricochet in the chest off the ribs or sternum, causing additional injury.

Compression

In a severe form of blunt trauma, the chest is rapidly and forcefully compressed, as by a steering wheel in a car crash or when something extremely heavy falls on the chest. The process is a sudden, severe compression of the chest, producing a rapid increase in intrathoracic pressure. Multiple fractures and flail chest can result. The increased intrathoracic pressure can cause the upper body to become swollen and cyanotic, the neck veins to distend, and the eyes appear to bulge.

Injury to the Back of the Chest

Direct blows to the back of the chest can cause contusions or rib fracture, along with spine and airway injury. Rarely, the scapula, which is protected by large muscles, receives a blow severe enough to fracture. When this happens, there may also be damage to the underlying chest wall and lung. Direct back blows to the lower rib cage can result in injuries to the spleen and kidneys.

INITIAL ASSESSMENT AND MANAGEMENT

First perform a primary survey with resuscitation of vital functions, then a detailed secondary survey, and finally definitive care. The basic tenant of chest trauma treatment identifies hypoxia as the most serious feature of chest injury and early interventions are designed to prevent or correct it. Life-threatening thoracic injuries are treated by airway control or an appropriately placed chest tube or needle. The secondary survey is influenced by a high index of suspicion for specific injuries.

CATEGORIES OF CHEST TRAUMA

Major thoracic injuries can be divided into two categories (see Table 7-1). Those injuries that are immediately life-threatening (lethal six) and those that can be difficult to diagnoses (hidden nine).

TABLE 7-1: MAJOR THORACIC INJURIES	
Lethal Six	**Hidden Nine**
Airway Obstruction	Rib Fractures
Open Pneumothorax	Sternal Fracture
Tension Pneumothorax	Pneumothorax
Flail Chest	Pulmonary Contusion
Massive Hemothorax	Esophageal Injury
Cardiac Tamponade	Tracheobronchial Disruption
	Diaphragmatic Rupture
	Blunt Cardiac Injury
	Aortic Rupture

Primary Survey: Life-threatening Injuries

Airway Obstruction

Control of airway is foremost in trauma care with simultaneous control of the cervical spine. The tongue is the most common cause of airway obstruction in the unconscious patient. Dentures, avulsed teeth, tissue, secretions, and blood can also contribute to airway obstruction. Bilateral mandibular fracture can also allow the tongue to collapse into the hypopharynx. Stridor, hoarseness, subcutaneous emphysema, altered mental status, accessory muscle use, apnea, and cyanosis are physical findings of airway obstruction. Immediately open the airway, suction as needed, and proceed toward oral intubation.

Open Pneumothorax/Sucking Chest Wound

Large defects of the chest wall result in an open pneumothorax or sucking chest wound. The severity of the open pneumothorax is related to the size of the wound opening. Stab wounds generally are self-sealing. A sucking, bubbling sound can sometimes be heard when examining the wound. Shotgun wounds are larger. If the opening is approximately two-thirds the diameter of the trachea, air will pass preferentially through the chest wall defect. This leads to ineffective ventilation, hypoxia, and hypercarbia.

Air entering through the wound remains in the pleural space. The lung does not expand. When the patient exhales, some air leaves through the wound. As the air moves in and out, the mediastinum moves with ventilation, compressing the opposite lung and great veins leading to the heart. The process of air moving in and out of an open chest wound makes a sucking sound.

First priority for a sucking chest wound is to apply a flutter dressing. This is a dry, nonocclusive 4" x 4" gauze dressing, taped on three sides, to allow air to escape but not to enter the wound. The patient must be closely monitored to ensure that a tension pneumothorax does not develop. If signs were to develop, immediate removal of the dressing is required.

Tension Pneumothorax

Tension pneumothorax is a minute-by-minute emergency. Prompt, correct, and efficient treatment will save a person's life. A pneumothorax becomes life threatening when the visceral pleura or a lung injury allows air to enter the pleural space and it cannot leave. The air leaks from the lung into the pleural space. Because the air is trapped in the pleural space, the space expands with every breath, compressing the lung to the point of complete collapse. The pressure in the affected side rises with each breath so that the collapsed lung presses against the heart and compresses the other lung.

As the pressure in the chest cavity increases, it may compress the vena cava, impairing blood return to the heart. The decrease in venous return to the heart decreases the cardiac output. If the mediastinal shift is great enough, the great vessels can become kinked sufficiently to prevent venous return to the heart. Death quickly follows.

Tension pneumothorax must have an intact, well-sealed chest to occur. But, it is not limited to closed-chest injuries. An open wound to the chest with a severe lung laceration can develop a tension pneumothorax after the wound has been sealed with gauze. The lung continues to leak air into a pleural space that is now sealed with the dressing; the pleural air cannot escape, causing a tension pneumothorax to develop.

Signs and Symptoms of Tension Pneumothorax

- Increasing difficulty breathing and shock due to the decreased flow of blood through the heart

- Respiratory distress

- Hypotension

- Tracheal deviation away from the injured side

- Absence of breath sounds on the injured side

- Neck vein distention

- Cyanosis or dusky color

- Hyperresonance on percussion of the injured side

- Asymmetry of chest wall motion

Tension pneumothorax is a clinical diagnosis and treatment should not be delayed by waiting for a chest x-ray. Management is to reduce the increasing pressure in the pleural space by removing the air.

Treatment of Tension Pneumothorax

- Rapidly insert a #14- or #16-gauge needle into the pleural space through the second intercostal space (over top of the 3rd rib).

- Immediately follow with a chest tube inserted into the 5th intercostal space (usually at nipple level) just anterior to the midaxillary line.

- If the tension pneumothorax occurs after an open wound has been bandaged, remove the dressing and reassess the patient.

- Cover open chest wounds with a flutter dressing.

- High flow oxygen per nonrebreather mask should also be administered.

Flail Chest

When three or more adjacent ribs are broken, each in two or more places, the part of the chest wall lying between the fractures becomes a free floating or flail segment (see Figure 7-2). The injury can also be a bilateral detachment of the sternum from the costal cartilage. Both types of injuries are most often the result of a massive crush injury or a high-speed motor crash. The loose segment collapses and does not expand with the chest wall during inhalation; it moves inward. During exhalation, the loose segment protrudes slightly while the rest of the chest wall contracts. Movement of the loose segment opposite to the normal movement of the chest wall is called **paradoxical movement** and looks uncoordinated with ventilatory actions. This paradoxical movement may not be visualized initially in the emergency department but may appear up to 12 to 16 hours after injury.

Flail chest is serious. It takes great force to cause a series of ribs to fracture in several places and produce flail chest. However, it is the lung contusion underlying the fractures that is of most concern. The lung under the segment does not expand properly during inhalation, which decreases the efficiency of ventilation. Chest radiograph may identify the rib fractures but initially miss the contusion. Chest computed tomography (CT) is most sensitive to identify pulmonary contusions and is often repeated after admission to monitor pulmonary contusion development.

Pulmonary contusion causes bleeding and swelling into the lung tissue. Pulmonary contusion often worsens over the first 36 hours after injury. As the contusion worsens there is loss of compliance, increased airway resistance, and decreased gas exchange. Hypoventilation followed by atelectasis, hypoxia, and cyanosis can occur. The patient should be followed carefully for respiratory failure. Prophylactic intubation is no longer endorsed. Liberal use of intercostal nerve blocks or epidural catheter insertion for analgesia administration along with aggressive pulmonary toilet and serial moni-

FIGURE 7-2: PARADOXICAL MOTION IN FLAIL CHEST

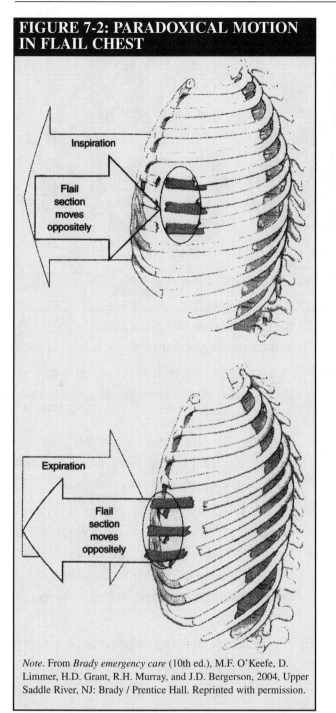

Note. From *Brady emergency care* (10th ed.), M.F. O'Keefe, D. Limmer, H.D. Grant, R.H. Murray, and J.D. Bergerson, 2004, Upper Saddle River, NJ: Brady / Prentice Hall. Reprinted with permission.

toring of blood gases will indicate whether the patient will ultimately require intubation and mechanical ventilation.

Massive Hemothorax

The presence of blood in the pleural space may occur in open or closed chest trauma and often accompanies pneumothorax (see Figure 7-3). Massive hemothorax results from a rapid accumulation of more than 1,500 ml of blood or one third or more of the patient's blood volume in the chest cavity. Blood comes from lacerated or torn vessels in the chest wall, bronchi, major vessels in the chest cavity, or a laceration of the lung. Common sites of major blood loss in the chest are laceration of the systemic or hilar vessels. Severe bleeding into the chest cavity causes hypovolemic shock.

Signs and Symptoms of Massive Hemothorax

• Absent breath sounds on the side of injury

• Asymmetry of chest wall motion with decreased movement on the side of injury

• Dullness to percussion on the side of injury

• Shock, hypotension, tachycardia

• Neck vein distention or flat neck veins

Treatment of Massive Hemothorax:

• Immediately insert chest tube.

• Fluid and blood volume resuscitation with large caliber IV lines.

• Blood from the chest tube may be collected and reinfused with an autotransfusion device (hospital specific).

• Notify surgeon of any continued chest bleeding of 200 ml/hr or more for 2 consecutive hours.

• Anticipate immediate thoracotomy when up to 1,200 to 1,500 ml of blood has been collected and the patient is hemodynamically unstable.

Cardiac Tamponade

Tamponade means pathologic compression. Pericardial tamponade is a rapidly progressive and life-threatening compression. The pericardium is a tough, fibrous, flexible but inelastic membrane surrounding the heart. As with the pleural space, there is a potential space with a small amount of fluid between the pericardium and the heart.

When the heart's blood vessels are damaged or if the myocardium is torn, blood enters the pericardial space. In the case of blunt trauma, there is no hole in the pericardium for the blood to empty from the space. With a gunshot wound, the hole in the

FIGURE 7-3: CONDITIONS PRODUCED BY CHEST INJURIES

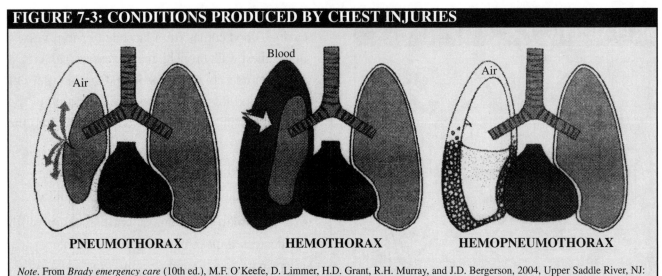

| PNEUMOTHORAX | HEMOTHORAX | HEMOPNEUMOTHORAX |

Note. From *Brady emergency care* (10th ed.), M.F. O'Keefe, D. Limmer, H.D. Grant, R.H. Murray, and J.D. Bergerson, 2004, Upper Saddle River, NJ: Brady/Prentice Hall. Reprinted with permission.

pericardium may or may not be large enough for the blood to drain from the pericardial space.

As the blood fills and cannot empty from the pericardial space, it rapidly begins to compress the heart because of the inelastic pericardium. The ventricles are squeezed, making it more difficult for the heart to refill. Thus, less blood is pumped out of the heart, and there is decreased cardiac output. Less and less blood gets pumped out with each contraction of the heart.

Initially, there may not be any symptoms other than those related to the chest injury. Because the pericardial sac is a fixed fibrous structure only a relatively small amount of blood is required to restrict cardiac activity and interfere with cardiac filling. Removal of small amounts of blood or fluid, often as little as 15 ml to 20 ml, by pericardiocentesis may result in immediate hemodynamic improvement.

<u>Signs and Symptoms of Cardiac Tamponade</u>

- Decreased systolic blood pressure

- Increased diastolic blood pressure

- Muffled heart tones

- Pulsus paradoxus is a decrease in systolic blood pressure greater then 10 mm Hg occuring during spontaneous inspiration

- Jugular vein distention occurring because the compressed ventricles cannot expand normally

to accommodate the blood entering the heart, venous pooling occurring in the head and neck

- Heart sounds may be distant sounding or muffled because the blood in the pericardium insulates the sound

- Hypotension occurring secondary to the myocardial compression and decreased cardiac output; shock progressively developing

- **Beck's Triad:** hypotension, muffled heart tones and distended neck veins are the classic signs of pericardial/cardiac tamponade however they occur with tamponade only in about 30% of the time (Peitzman, Rhodes, Schwab, Yealy, & Fabian, 2002)

- Associated injuries and problems such as hypovolemia may mask the triad of symptoms

- Insertion of a central venous line and elevated pressure are also diagnostic

- As tamponade progresses, the patient develops air hunger, becomes agitated, and his level of consciousness decreases

- Pulseless electrical activity (PEA) in the absence of hypovolemia and tension pneumothorax suggests cardiac tamponade.

<u>Treatment of Cardiac Tamponade</u>

- Assist with focused assessment sonogram in

trauma (FAST) exam, which is an ultrasound of the heart. This can be performed rapidly in the emergency department and may be 90% accurate for the presence of pericardial fluid (Peitzman et al., 2002). It is however operator skill dependent.

- Assist with needle pericardiocentesis, the insertion of a needle into the pericardium to drain the blood. This is diagnostic as well as therapeutic, but it is still not definitive.

- Prepare the patient for the operating room for a thoracotomy, pericardiotomy, and repair of the injured heart.

Resuscitative Emergency Department Thoracotomy

Closed chest cardiopulmonary resuscitation for cardiac arrest or PEA is generally ineffective in a hypovolemic bleeding patient with penetrating chest wounds. Penetrating thoracic injury patients who arrive pulseless, but with myocardial electrical activity, may be candidates for immediate emergency department thoracotomy. A surgeon must be present at the time of the patient's arrival to determine the potential success of this controversial maneuver. A left anterior thoracotomy is performed to gain access. Restoration of intravascular volume is continued, and endotracheal intubation and mechanical ventilation are essential. The highest survival rates are in patients with cardiac stab wounds who suddenly arrest from pericardial tamponade (Moore et al., 2004). Nurses must quickly set up an open thoracotomy tray with rib spreaders as well as ensuring that universal precautions are in place. Aggressive fluid resuscitation ensues with crystalloid and blood products as well as timely notification of the operating room for impending arrival.

Secondary Survey: Life-threatening Chest Injuries

Rib Fracture

Frequently seen, rib fractures are most often caused by direct blunt, compression, or crush injury.

Car crashes and falls in older adults are common mechanisms of injury. The fractures may be single or multiple.

It should be assumed that injury to the clavicle or above involves closed-head injury, neck injury, and facial fractures. The upper ribs are considered the first three ribs which are strong, protected by the shoulder girdle, and not as likely to be fractured. A fracture to the upper ribs indicates a powerful blow and possible accompanying serious head and neck injury. In addition, suspect trauma to the subclavian vein or aorta. Fractures to the upper ribs carry a high mortality related to the injury of the underlying structures.

The middle ribs refer to the middle six ribs (4th through 9th), which are most likely to sustain a fracture. The lower ribs refer to the last three ribs (10th through 12th). Maintain a high index of suspicion for liver and spleen injuries for patients with lower right-sided and left-sided rib fractures respectively.

Rib Fracture Signs and Symptoms

There may be deformity and contusion or laceration at the injured site. Deep breathing and movement is usually painful, so the patient will take shallow breaths and lean toward the side of the injury. Respiratory rate and patterns should be assessed to evaluate the injury's impact on ventilation. Pain management is important and may require epidural anesthesia or intercostal nerve blocks. Good pulmonary toilet of coughing, incentive spirometry, and deep breathing is essential to prevent pneumonia or atelectasis. Occasionally, the end of a fractured rib punctures or tears a lung or the chest wall, causing a hemothorax or pneumothorax.

Sternal Fracture

Enormous anterior chest impact is necessary to fracture the sternum, such as occurs with a steering wheel. There is a significant possibility for blunt cardiac injury. Chest CT and electrocardiograms (ECGs) are routinely performed with all steering-wheel injuries to the chest to detect blunt cardiac injury.

Pneumothorax

A simple pneumothorax is the presence of air in the pleural space. The source of air can be external through an open chest wound or from a laceration of the lung tissue, such as by a fractured rib, or a ruptured lung. The air separates the parietal and visceral pleura and collects in the pleural space, causing the lung to collapse. As air pressure in the pleural space increases, the lung collapses further and may fully collapse. Air can also accumulate in the mediastinum. In the case where the chest wall defect is small, the body is sometimes able to reseal itself.

The patient will complain of shortness of breath and pain. Breath sounds are diminished on the affected side. Tachycardia and tachypnea are usually evident.

Placement of a chest tube connected to underwater drainage (in the 4th or 5th intercostal space) is the treatment of choice to reexpand the lung. The patient should be in a semi-Fowler's position to prevent pressure against the diaphragm from the abdominal organs. High-flow oxygen is administered. The patient should be monitored constantly for the development of tension pneumothorax. A chest tube should be placed prior to transporting the patient with a pneumothorax via air ambulance.

Pulmonary Contusion

Pulmonary contusion is defined as traumatic lung parenchymal damage with edema and hemorrhage without lung laceration. Injury to lung parenchyma becomes progressively worse because of rupture and bleeding into the lung tissue, alveoli, and small airways. The airways collapse and ventilation is lost, resulting in hypoxemia. As inflammatory response develops, gas exchange is impaired and the patient's condition worsens. Therefore, respiratory failure may be subtle and develops over time rather than occurring instantaneously.

Pulmonary contusion severity peaks at 48 to 72 hours postinjury. Careful monitoring and reevaluation of the patient is warranted. Pulse oximetry monitoring, arterial blood gas determinations, ECG monitoring, and appropriate ventilatory equipment are necessary for optimal management.

Dyspnea, hemoptysis, hypoxia, and possible chest wall ecchymosis or abrasions are present in the clinical picture. Whenever a patient has a history of chest trauma, pulmonary contusion should be suspected and looked for. Patients sustaining pulmonary contusion may exhibit external physical findings. Chest x-ray does not always identify a pulmonary contusion while CT scan is highly diagnostic. Patients with significant hypoxia should be intubated and ventilated within the first hour after injury.

Esophageal Injury

Esophageal injuries are infrequent and deadly. Most often penetration is the cause of injury, but a severe blow to the lower abdomen can disrupt the esophagus. Other causes are accidental damage from an instrument during a procedure, caustic ingestion, crush injury, and blast injury.

Esophageal injuries can cause mediastinitis from contamination by saliva and gastric contents and may ultimately lead to empyema.

Esophageal injury should be suspected:

1. When a patient who received a severe blow to the lower sternum or epigsastrium shows evidence of severe shock and pain disproportionate to the apparent injury

2. When there is a left pneumothorax or hemothorax without associated rib fractures

3. When particulate matter appears in the chest tube after blood begins to clear

4. Presence of mediastinal air as confirmed by esophagram.

Esophageal injury requires urgent diagnosis and surgical repair. Delays to identification lead to further complications and prolonged length of hospitalization.

Tracheobronchial Disruption

Major injuries to the trachea or bronchi are caused by blunt or penetrating trauma to the neck and chest and are frequently overlooked, as there are many associated injuries to this area. As a consequence of delayed or missed diagnosis, there is a high mortality rate. There may be massive crepitus from the nipples up, frothy or bloody sputum in the airway, and noisy breathing. Complete obstruction may take place.

Any point of the tracheobronchial tree can be damaged with blunt or penetrating trauma. Because of proximity to major blood vessels, injury can cause exsanguinating hemorrhage into the chest and mediastinum or into the airway itself, producing asphyxia. Signs are severe dyspnea, hemoptysis, subcutaneous emphysema, mediastinal crunch, or tension pneumothorax. A pneumothorax associated with a persistent large air leak after tube thoracostomy suggests a tracheobronchial injury until proven otherwise. More than one chest tube may be necessary to overcome a large air leak and expand the lung. The patient may have dyspnea, tachycardia, and diminished or absent breath sounds. Airway support may be adequate until inflammation and edema resolve, but surgery is necessary if the tear is significant or healing fails to occur.

Diaphragmatic Rupture

A traumatic diaphragmatic rupture is more commonly diagnosed on the left side. It is thought that the liver hides or protects the defect on the right side. In penetrating injuries, herniation may take years to manifest. Hemothorax, pneumothorax, or intra-abdominal bleeding raise a flag to look for a ruptured diaphragm. Large tears may cause herniation of abdominal contents into the thorax. The nasogastric tube may be seen on the chest x-ray. Other indicators are dyspnea, decreased breath sounds on the affected side, abdominal or epigastric pain radiating to the left shoulder, or bowel sounds in the lower chest. Direct operative repair of diaphragmatic injuries is necessary.

Blunt Cardiac Injury

Blunt trauma to the anterior chest from steering wheels, falls, assaults, and other direct blows can bruise the heart. Signs and symptoms are not specific to the injury. History of significant blunt trauma to the chest is an important indicator. However, the patient may not display an indication of chest wall injury. Chest pain, abrasions, and contusions to the chest and fractures are all seen in other chest injuries. Chest pain in blunt cardiac injury (BCI) is similar to angina, but does not clear with the use of coronary vasodilators.

Mild BCI can have a dysrhythmia and normal echocardiogram. Severe BCI while rare can mimic an acute myocardial infarction and will demonstrate abnormalities on echocardiogram. Patients presenting with dysrhythmias require at least 12 to 24 hours of further telemetry monitoring. Common dysrhythmias include sinus tachycardia, atrial fibrillation, and premature ventricular contractions (PVCs). Echocardiogram is helpful in determining the degree of myocardial wall dyskinesia or abnormal other wall motion abnormalities.

Historically cardiac enzymes, specifically CK-MB (released into the bloodsteam with cardiac muscle injury), were used to detect blunt myocardial injury. However, most trials revealed that CK-MB does not correlate with myocardial injury (Ferrera et al., 2001). Cardiac troponins may diagnose myocardial infarction, however their use in diagnosing blunt cardiac injury is inconclusive and offers no additional information. Therefore cardiac enzymes have no role in the evaluation and management of the patient with blunt cardiac injury (Ferrera et al., 2001).

Aortic Rupture

Traumatic aortic rupture is usually caused by a severe deceleration injury from a motor vehicle crash or a fall from great height. The heart and aortic arch suddenly move forward causing shearing at the point of the aorta's attachment to the heart. Of these injuries, 80% result in free rupture and have complete exsanguination into the pleural space in the first hour (Peitzman et al., 2002). For those that survive immediately, salvage is frequently possible if aortic rupture is identified and treated early. In a very few, the tear is small and covered over by the outer fibrous layer of the aorta. This covering over will last for only a brief time and then give away. The patient will then bleed out.

Specific signs and symptoms are frequently absent. A high index of suspicion prompted by a history of decelerating force and characteristic radiologic findings followed by arteriography help make the diagnosis.

The following signs on initial chest x-ray should prompt further evaluation:

1. Widened mediastinum

2. Obliteration of the aortic knob

3. Deviation of the trachea or esophagus to the right

4. Fractures of the first or second rib or scapula

If there is the slightest suspicion of aortic injury, the patient should be evaluated at a hospital capable of repairing the injury.

<u>Diagnostic Tests for Aortic Tear</u>

Aortogram

Aortography versus chest computed tomography (CT) is debated as the best diagnostic test for diagnosis of aortic tear. The aortogram remains the gold standard in the diagnosis of blunt aortic rupture. Aortogram defines anatomy preoperatively and helps determine the need for cardiopulmonary bypass for ascending aortic injuries and identifies multiple tears, which occur in up to 20% of aortic injuries (Scaletta & Schaider, 2001).

Helical CT

Helical CT of the chest is rapidly gaining favor as the diagnostic test of choice and has been shown to be an accurate rapid screening method for patients with suspected blunt aortic injury, in many large Level I trauma centers. Chest CT however, is dependent upon the grade of CT scanner available and the expertise of the radiologist performing the study. Not all hospitals have recent high-end helical CT scanners or available highly trained radiologists, therefore, angiography should be used as an alternative.

Transesophageal Echocardiography

Transesophageal echocardiography (TEE) is recommended in unstable patients with clinical suspicion of aortic tear. TEE is an effective diagnostic ultrasound test that allows a look at the heart muscle and blood flow from a tube that is passed into the esophagus. The benefit of TEE is that it is portable, noninvasive, and rapid. It is a useful alternative to angiogram when hospitals have difficulty obtaining aortography, particularly at night and on weekends. Results, however, are dependent upon operator skill.

ASSESSMENT

The effectiveness of thoracic trauma care is directly related to the patient's ability to breathe. Initial assessment is directed to airway and ventilation, the standard ABC assessment. Assume head and neck injury until the patient's airway is cleared. The upper airway must be cleared and maintained. Ventilation support and oxygen should be given if the patient has respiratory distress and before further assessment is conducted.

Thoracic trauma often includes multiple injuries. Patient history and knowledge of the mechanism of injury are important in determining the full scope of damage to the patient. Knowing the object causing the trauma, the speed of the force, and the physical site of initial injury is essential information. If you are in the prehospital setting, gather information from the scene, the patient, and bystanders. If you are in the emergency department, be sure to get a full report and documentation from EMS and the patient (if possible).

Patients with obvious or suspected chest injuries must be immediately and quickly assessed in an organized and thorough manner, followed by rapid essential interventions. Speed in assessment is essential.

THORACIC ASSESSMENT OVERVIEW

- Impaled object in chest

- Open wound into the chest

- Signs of tension pneumothorax after a dressing is applied

- Obvious deformity of the chest wall, rib cage, or neck; trachea displaced from the midline

- Unequal chest expansion

- Paradoxical movement of flail chest

- Labored breathing (rate, depth, and effort)

- Decreased breath sounds on the affected side

- Hemoptysis, signs of hemorrhagic shock

- Hypoventilation and splinting of the injured side

- Air hunger, agitation, and decreased level of consciousness

- Hypotension, muffled heart sounds, and distended neck veins

- Weak rapid pulse with falling blood pressure

- Bulging of the tissues of the chest wall between the ribs and above the clavicle

- Cyanosis of the face and neck

- Sucking chest wound

- Identify subcutaneous emphysema by palpating for a crackling in the subcutaneous tissues

INTERVENTIONS

Although there are many types of chest injuries, the same principles of care apply to all of them:

- Rapidly conduct the ABCs, open and maintain the airway, and stabilize breathing and circulation.

- Assess the patient's breathing rate, depth, and effort after the airway is open and maintained.

- Apply supplemental oxygen; provide respiratory support when necessary.

- Be prepared for life-threatening hypovolemic shock. Two large-bore IV catheters should be immediately inserted for warmed fluid resuscitation, and high-flow oxygen should be administered.

- Observe and palpate neck veins for distention, which can indicate compression or obstruction of return blood flow to the heart.

- Promptly apply three-sided flutter dressings to open chest wounds and monitor for the development of tension pneumothorax.

- Relieve signs and symptoms of a tension pneumothorax by loosening one side of the dressing on the wound. If it is a closed chest injury, assist with the placement of a large-bore needle into the pleural space.

- Palpate the chest wall for symmetry of chest wall movement, structural deformities, crepitus, subcutaneous emphysema, or point tenderness.

- Observe, monitor, and record vital signs serially; check for bilateral and equal breath sounds.

- Compare the findings of the vital sign measurements with the appearance of the patient's condition to see if they appear consistent.

- Monitor ECG and look for arrhythmia.

- Assist with positive pressure bag-mask ventilation.

- Control bleeding from the chest wall with direct pressure.

- Stabilize impaled objects to minimize movement. **Never remove impaled objects.**

- Prepare for emergency thoracotomy for the following indications:

  - Massive hemothorax (> 1,500 ml blood returned on insertion of chest tube)

  - Ongoing bleeding from chest > 200 ml/hr for 2 or more hours

  - Suspicion of cardiac tamponade

  - Acute deterioration from penetrating transmediastinal chest wounds

- Chest wall disruption

- Radiographic evidence of great vessel injury

- Suspected air embolism

- Impalement wounds to the chest

SUMMARY

Thoracic injuries account for 25% of all trauma deaths annually in the United States (Peitzman et al., 2002). Thoracic trauma is high risk because of the vital organs in the chest and the high potential for respiratory impediment. There is a high incidence of other injuries associated with chest trauma. Chest injuries are common in multiple system trauma and are associated with life-threatening problems, both from the direct trauma and the resulting complications.

Organized, rapid assessment and intervention is essential, as is the ability to recognize acute signs and symptoms specific to thoracic trauma. Despite the many types of thoracic injuries, almost all require the same initial care. The aim of emergency care is directly related to the patient's ability to ventilate effectively. The body cannot store oxygen and needs a continuous supply. Any injury to the chest requires evaluation as serious trauma.

Internal bleeding from lacerations to the chest organs and major blood vessels is potentially deadly. Hemorrhaging can compress the lungs and vessels. A few minutes are often all that separates the patient from life or death.

EXAM QUESTIONS

CHAPTER 7

Questions 44-49

44. Decreased breath sounds and asymmetry of chest wall motion on one side could result from

    a. abnormal anatomy.

    b. pericardial tamponade.

    c. cardiac contusion.

    d. tension pneumothorax.

45. Which of the following signs and symptoms would differentiate cardiac tamponade from tension pneumothorax?

    a. Tachycardia

    b. Absent unilateral breath sounds

    c. Narrowed pulse pressure

    d. Jugular venous distention

46. Which injury is characterized by Beck's triad of hypotension, muffled heart sounds, and distended neck veins?

    a. Sucking chest wound

    b. Tension pneumothorax

    c. Hemopneumothorax

    d. Pericardial tamponade

47. A 42-year-old man sustains multiple rib fractures as a result of a tractor rollover. Emergency department examination reveals a flail chest. The patient is receiving oxygen via nonrebreather mask and IV lactated Ringer's solution. The patient exhibits progressive confusion, cyanosis, and tachypnea. The priority nursing intervention to take is

    a. prepare for endotracheal intubation and mechanical ventilation.

    b. IV sedation.

    c. external stabilization of the chest wall.

    d. prepare for administration of intercostal nerve blocks.

48. Which of the following is indicated for the immediate management of an open pneumothorax?

    a. Cricothyroidotomy

    b. Flutter dressing

    c. Needle chest decompression

    d. Positive pressure ventilation

49. Emergency open thoracotomy performed in the emergency department may be indicated for

    a. cold water drowning.

    b. stab wound to the heart.

    c. crush injury to the heart.

    d. motor vehicle crash.

CHAPTER 8

ABDOMINAL TRAUMA

CHAPTER OBJECTIVE

Upon completion of this chapter, the reader will be able to describe the key components of managing abdominal trauma.

LEARNING OBJECTIVES

Upon completion of this chapter, the reader should be able to

1. choose appropriate physical assessment skills used to identify abdominal injuries.

2. describe common mechanisms of injury to the abdomen.

3. recognize characteristics of common abdominal injuries.

4. identify the appropriate diagnostic test to identify abdominal injuries.

INTRODUCTION

Abdominal trauma is probably one of the most frequently overlooked or missed groups of injuries. Life-threatening abdominal injuries may not have any outward sign of trauma. When the injuries are undetected, they have a high potential for causing death.

Motor vehicle crashes (MVCs) cause approximately 75% of the blunt abdominal injuries (Peitzman et al., 2002). Falls, other types of vehicular crashes (such as bicycles or motorcycles), sports, and assaults account for most of the other mechanisms of abdominal trauma.

Patients involved in high-energy blunt injury have multiple problems that are particularly difficult to assess. They are often intoxicated, have closed-head injuries, and tend to have multisystem trauma. Reliable abdominal examination is confounded by several variables. These include presence of distracting injury, presence of spinal cord injury, altered level of consciousness, and influence of drugs and alcohol.

MECHANISM OF INJURY

As with other trauma, mechanisms of abdominal injury, blunt or penetrating, may be closed or open. Intra-abdominal injuries can result from three different mechanisms. One method is compression causing a crush injury. A second method is from an abrupt shearing force causing tears of organs or vascular supply. A third method is from a sudden rise in intra-abdominal pressure causing rupture of an intra-abdominal viscus. Table 8-1 reveals that the spleen, liver, and small bowel are the most commonly injured abdominal organs in blunt trauma while the liver, small bowel, diaphragm, and colon are the most commonly injured abdominal organs in penetrating trauma (American College of Surgeons, 2004a).

TABLE 8-1: ABDOMINAL ORGANS MOST FREQUENTLY INJURED IN DECREASING INCIDENCE

Blunt Trauma	Penetrating Trauma
Spleen	Liver
Liver	Small bowel
Small bowel	Diaphragm
	Colon

CLOSED BLUNT INJURY

When the abdomen receives a severe blow, usually from deceleration or compression, as with a steering wheel, sports injury, or assault, it is considered a closed blunt injury.

Remember that blunt abdominal injury is deceptive because damage can be severe, even life-threatening, without immediate outward signs. Vital functions must be watched closely for changes in the patient's condition as indicators of unseen problems. If there is massive hemorrhage into the abdomen, there may be a blue-gray discoloration around the umbilicus; however, most often there is little visible evidence.

In compression incidents, the organs are crushed between solid objects, for instance, the steering wheel and spinal column. Along with direct damage, the organs are often pushed out of place, resulting in additional injuries such as herniation of the diaphragm.

Deceleration events may rupture solid organs or vessels in the abdominal cavity because of tearing forces exerted against stabilizing ligaments and the vessels. When hollow organs are ruptured or lacerated, their contents will spill into the peritoneal cavity, causing an inflammatory reaction. Solid organs have a large blood supply subject to hemorrhage, which is also seen in the rupture of major vessels. Pelvic fractures causing bladder and urethral injuries may lead to hemorrhage and life-threatening conditions. Loss of blood into the abdominal cavity can contribute to hypovolemic shock.

Blunt trauma from a MVC is influenced by where the patient is sitting, speed of the vehicle, use and type of seat belt, air bag deployment, and whether there was ejection from the vehicle. Although seat belt use has decreased fatalities, it can also cause injuries to the colon, small bowel, stomach, liver, spleen, vascular structures, and spinal cord.

Injuries from falls vary with the height of the fall, landing surface, and part of the body that hits the surface first.

OPEN PENETRATING INJURY

Open penetrating injuries range from a slight laceration of the abdominal wall to deep penetration through the peritoneum into the abdominal cavity. It may be difficult to determine if the wound extends into the abdominal cavity, but in the case of stabbing or gunshot wounds, it should be assumed the peritoneum has been penetrated.

The depth of injury may be deceptive; while appearing minimal, it can be devastating. Multiple organ damage is likely in the case of gunshot wounds. A clean, little bullet hole may cause torn vessels and tissue beneath. Stab wounds are often self-contained because they have less velocity.

It should also be noted that the diaphragm extends to the 4th intercostal space during exhalation, and penetrating injuries into the thorax may also involve the abdomen. Penetrating wounds into the flank or buttocks can also enter the abdominal cavity, hitting a major vessel, a segment of the bowel, or a solid organ.

Most penetrating injuries are caused by projectiles and are intentionally inflicted. These wounds imply violence, especially as violence escalates in this country. Damage includes laceration, impalement, puncture, and rupture.

The cause of the injury should be identified. In the case of a gunshot, the type of gun, caliber, proximity to the patient when fired, and number of shots that hit the patient are important in determining the likely extent of injury. It is necessary to identify the length, width, and composition of other penetrating objects as well. Injuries from wood are likely to cause infection because it is a biologic material.

Evisceration is the result of an extensive laceration of the abdominal wall that causes the organs to protrude through the wound. The organs should not be pushed back into the abdomen but instead covered with a moist, sterile dressing. It is essential that the organs are kept warm and moist. Dressings should not be a material that clings or loses substance when wet, such as tissuelike paper.

Impalement injuries vary with the type of object lodged in the abdomen and the structures that are damaged. The impaled object often compresses and tamponades affected organs and vessels, which acts to hold back hemorrhaging. Therefore, the impaled object should not be removed. Secure the object in place until medical management determines the mode of treatment.

Genitourinary trauma comprises only a small percent of trauma cases. The anatomical location of the structures and organs make life-threatening injuries infrequent. Trauma occurs most often to the kidneys or bladder. Because the bladder is hollow, it is more likely to be seriously damaged when full and distended, than when empty and collapsible.

As with the intra-abdominal injuries in the peritoneal cavity, organs and structures injured in the retroperitoneal space are difficult to immediately assess for damage. Injuries are usually not isolated to a particular organ but in association with multiple injuries. It takes such force to damage a kidney that this injury is usually in association with a fractured rib or other intra-abdominal injuries. A patient with multiple injuries involving the lower abdomen or pelvis should always be considered to have a good

probability for renal damage. Blunt injury is the most common mechanism in urologic trauma.

BLUNT MECHANISMS

Blunt mechanisms are the most common of all urologic injuries, accounting for 70-80% of the trauma (Peitzman et al., 2002). Examples of blunt mechanisms are motor vehicle deceleration impact; falls; objects, such as a bat or fist striking the flank or external genitalia; blunt force strong enough to fracture the pelvis and cause damage to the bladder and urethra; and rape.

Blunt trauma to the back or flank related to kidney damage is most often a simple self-healing renal contusion. In cases of severe lower abdominal injury or pelvic fracture, urologic damage should always be considered. If the trauma is severe, the kidney will fracture.

OVERVIEW OF ANATOMY AND PHYSIOLOGY AND SPECIFIC ORGAN INJURY PATTERNS

The abdominal cavity is one of two body cavities, the other being the thoracic cavity. The diaphragm separates the two cavities (see Figure 8-1).

Diaphragm

Ninety percent of diaphragmatic injuries are associated with high-speed MVCs (Peitzman et al., 2002). Diaphragm injury may accompany, and should always be suspected, in thoracic or abdominal blunt and penetrating trauma. The injury can be easily overlooked. Diaphragmatic rupture occurs equally on the right and left sides, but is more readily identified on the left side because the liver prevents the abdominal contents from herniating into the chest on the right side.

If the diaphragm is lacerated, the abdominal contents will enter the chest cavity, causing

FIGURE 8-1: INTRATHORACIC ABDOMEN

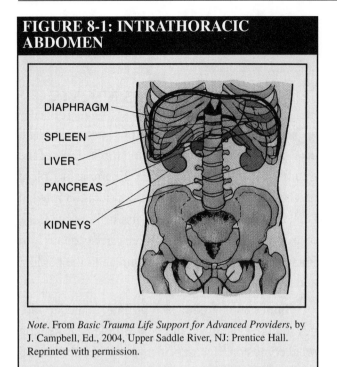

DIAPHRAGM

SPLEEN

LIVER

PANCREAS

KIDNEYS

Note. From *Basic Trauma Life Support for Advanced Providers*, by J. Campbell, Ed., 2004, Upper Saddle River, NJ: Prentice Hall. Reprinted with permission.

TABLE 8-2: THE TWO ABDOMINAL SPACES

Peritoneal Space	Retroperitoneal Space
• Bowel	• Abdominal aorta
• Gallbladder	• Bladder
• Liver	• Inferior vena cava
• Pancreas	• Kidneys
• Spleen	• Reproductive organs
• Stomach	• Ureters

impaired breathing due to lung compression and the loss of negative pressure. Signs and symptoms include decreased breath sounds on the affected side and complaints of dyspnea and cyanosis. There may be a shift in heart sounds. Bowel sounds may be heard in the hemithorax. Diagnosis is confirmed by chest x-ray or during surgery for another traumatic repair. A hemopneumothorax may also be evident. Immediate surgical intervention is required.

Beginning below the diaphragm, the abdominal cavity extends down to the pubic area. It is bounded by the spine in the back and the ribs and abdominal muscle wall in the front. When referring to descriptive geographic areas of the abdomen, it is thought of as being divided into quadrants: left and right upper quadrants and left and right lower quadrants.

Within the abdomen there are two spaces: the peritoneal space and retroperitoneal space. They contain the major organs of the digestive, endocrine, and urogenital systems, along with major blood vessels (see Table 8-2).

The mesentery, also called greater and lesser omentum, is formed from the peritoneum and carries blood vessels and nerves to the abdominal organs. It is a fold forming a sheet of fragile tissue that surrounds organs and suspends them from the body wall. The structure of the omentum allows the organs to hang freely, permitting movement within the abdominal cavity.

The abdominal organs or viscus are considered to be hollow, solid, or vascular. Hollow organs are tubes that conduct or store material, such as food being stored in and moved through the stomach or urine being stored in the bladder. Hollow organs do not bleed as much as solid organs do. Hollow organs include the stomach, duodenum, small and large intestine, appendix, rectum, gallbladder, bile ducts, urinary bladder, ureters, and uterus.

Solid organs are masses of tissue where much of the body's chemical work takes place. They include the liver, spleen, pancreas, kidneys, ovaries, and adrenal glands. Vascular organs are masses of tissue rich in blood vessels such as the liver, kidneys, and spleen.

Solid organs fracture when injured; hollow organs rupture or collapse. Solid and vascular structures bleed, while hollow organs empty their contents. The consequences can be intra-abdominal bleeding, peritonitis, and sepsis.

Major vascular structures supplying the abdomen are the abdominal aorta that bifurcates into the iliac arteries (to supply the lower extremities), the celiac trunk, and the inferior and superior mesentery arteries that supply the abdomen. The inferior vena cava is formed by the union of two common iliac veins and is the major vein in the abdomen.

ORGANS

Peritoneal Space

Stomach

The stomach is a hollow organ in the left upper quadrant that is protected by the lower left ribs. Stomach size changes with the amount of contents, and when empty, is more able to compress and absorb energy during trauma. Blunt gastric injuries are rare, while gastric injury occurs in about 15% of penetrating trauma (Peitzman et al., 2002). The stomach has an extensive blood supply, so hematemesis and blood in the nasogastric aspirate are likely when the stomach is injured. Subdiaphragmatic air may be seen on a chest x-ray in blunt gastric rupture. Surgical exploration and intervention is required.

Small Bowel

The small bowel or intestine is a large hollow organ and has three sections: the duodenum, jejunum, and ileum. Hanging from its mesentery, the small bowel lies entirely free within the abdomen and is approximately seven meters long. This part of the mesentery contains arteries branching from the aorta and veins that carry blood to the liver. The small bowel is one of the most commonly injured abdominal organs in penetrating trauma; blunt mechanism of injury is less common.

Small perforations can occur from blowouts of closed loops (seat belt injuries) whereas larger perforations are caused by direct blows or shearing injury.

Small bowel injury should be considered when there is bruising from a lap belt (seat belt sign). There may also be an associated fracture of the lumbar spine known as a Chance fracture. Small bowel injury is not usually identified on computed tomography CT scan. Therefore a high index of suspicion along with clinical symptoms of increasing abdominal pain and increasing white blood cell count will prompt the surgeon to operate. Delayed diagnosis of

small bowel injury greater than 24 hours is related to increased morbidity and mortality.

Colon and Rectum

Also a major hollow organ, the large intestine interfaces with the small intestine proximally and ends at the rectum. About 5-feet long, the large intestine lies around the border of the small bowel. It has three sections called the cecum, colon, and rectum. The primary function is to absorb the remaining 5% to 10% of the fluid from the contents and form stool.

Colon damage is seen in about one quarter of the gunshot and stabbing wounds to the abdomen (Peitzman et al., 2002). Only a small percentage of colon injuries are caused by blunt mechanisms. Rectal injuries are a small percentage of the colon injuries, but blunt rectal perforation can be associated with pelvic fractures, concussion (explosion) injuries, devascularization from a mesentery injury, or foreign objects. Gross rectal bleeding may indicate a pelvic fracture damaging the colon or rectum.

Liver

The liver is the largest organ in the body, weighing almost 3% of the total body weight and is located in the upper right quadrant of the abdomen. The liver is extremely vascular, essentially being a large, dense mass of blood vessels and cells. All of the blood pumped to the gastrointestinal (GI) tract is pumped through the liver before returning to the heart.

The location of the liver makes it vulnerable to trauma, more likely from penetrating than blunt mechanisms. Usually liver injuries are not fatal. The liver is encapsulated by a tough fibrous sheath and is vascular. Injury may only affect the capsule, or cause a contused, lacerated, or fractured liver.

Ultrasound of the abdomen will increase the potential for correct diagnosis. Right rib fractures or a blow to the right upper quadrant should raise an alert to liver damage. Most likely, there is pain and tenderness in the area of the liver, to the point of guarding, along with bruising and nausea. If the damage is severe, there will be hemodynamic instability.

Gallbladder

The liver's connection to the intestine is the bile duct. The gallbladder is an out pouching of the bile duct and a reservoir for bile. Trauma to the gallbladder is rare.

Spleen

The primary function of the spleen is immunologic, for example, the production and destruction of blood cells, but it is not necessary to sustain life. If removed, the spleen's functions are taken over by the liver and bone marrow. As little as 20-25% of the remaining spleen can provide immunologic function if part of the spleen is to be removed (Peitzman et al., 2002).

The spleen, located in the left upper quadrant, just beneath the diaphragm and in front of the lower ribs, is a major solid organ, smaller than the liver. The largest mass of lymphatic tissue in the body, the spleen is vascular and enclosed in a capsule supported by three ligaments. Although the ribs protect the spleen, the ligaments can be torn from the spleen in blunt injury, causing severe hemorrhage.

Although the spleen is relatively small and not likely to be injured by penetrating trauma, it is the number one most commonly injured abdominal organ from blunt trauma (American College of Surgeons, 2004b). Blunt trauma is usually the result of compression or deceleration force seen in MVCs, falls, or direct blows to the abdomen. Like the liver, the spleen is encapsulated. A splenic injury can affect just the capsule or cause a hematoma, laceration, or fracture.

Injury to the left upper quadrant and lower ribs is likely to include the spleen. There may be pain in the left upper quadrant or referred to the left shoulder, also known as Kehr's sign. Bruising and signs of hypovolemia with tachycardia and hypotension may be apparent. Physical examination is not specific for splenic trauma. In an unstable patient, an ultrasound will provide the most rapid diagnosis of hemoperitoneum, a frequent consequence of trauma.

If the spleen is ruptured, or there is a penetrating wound that causes severe hemorrhage, the patient could exsanguinate rapidly without immediate surgical intervention. Management depends on the hemodynamic stability of the patient, age, associated injuries, the degree of hemoperitoneum, and the severity of the splenic injury. Nonoperative management of spleen injuries is now the norm. However, for the patient to be observed, it should be done in a facility with rapid access to the CT scanner, a surgeon, and the operating room.

Pancreas

The pancreas is a flat, solid, firmly fixed organ, lying deep in the abdomen behind the stomach, below the liver, and in front of the 1st and 2nd lumbar vertebrae. Its head is attached to the duodenum and the tail reaches to the spleen. Penetrating trauma to the pancreas is more common than blunt injury. Blunt injury, however, is more common in children resulting from crush injury between the spine and another object, such as a steering wheel or handle bar.

Diagnosis is based on the mechanism of injury and the high rate of associated intra-abdominal injury. Pancreatic injuries are rarely isolated. If the injury is confined to the pancreas, signs initially may be nonspecific. Within 24 hr of the injury, the patient will complain of midepigastric or back pain. Often, a laparotomy is necessary to confirm the pancreatic damage and to repair other abdominal injuries. When surgery is necessary, major efforts are made to save the pancreas because of its vital endocrine and exocrine functions.

Retroperitoneal Space

Behind the peritoneum and outside the peritoneal cavity is the retroperitoneal space. It contains the abdominal aorta, bladder, inferior vena cava, kidneys, reproductive organs, and ureters.

Kidneys

The kidneys lie in a fatty tissue layer on the left and right side of the posterior wall of the abdomen, just above the waist at the costovertebral angle. They are enclosed in a strong fibrous capsule. The kidneys are well protected by the vertebrae and muscles of the back and abdominal viscera in the front. Kidneys are highly vascular; nearly 20% of the cardiac output passes through them every minute. Of renal injuries, 80% are from blunt trauma resulting in a loss of kidney in 5%, whereas the kidney loss in penetrating trauma is twice as high (Peitzman et al., 2002).

Ureters

Small flexible muscular tubes, the ureters drain the urine from each kidney into the bladder. The ureters are so well protected, lying deep in the retroperitoneal space, that they are rarely injured from blunt trauma. Most ureteral injuries are from penetrating trauma, mainly gunshot wounds.

Urinary Bladder

The urinary bladder is supported by ligaments and protected behind the symphysis pubis in the pelvic cavity. Ureters enter at the base posteriorly at each side of the bladder. Urine capacity ordinarily is about 500 ml and emptying occurs through the urethra. The bladder has an abundant blood supply, primarily from branches of the internal iliac artery.

Most bladder ruptures are from blunt trauma; 80% are extraperitoneal and 20% are intraperitoneal (Peitzman et al., 2002). Extraperitoneal rupture is generally caused by pelvic fracture. Intraperitoneal rupture is associated with a full bladder at the time of impact.

Urethra

In the male, the urethra is about 8 in. (20 cm) long and passes through the penis on the exterior of the body. In the female, the urethra is short, about 1.5 in. (3.8 cm). Protected internally by the symphysis pubis, the woman's urethra opens in front of the vagina. The mechanism of urethral injury is usually blunt and is often associated with pelvic fractures or straddle injuries.

Pelvic Fracture

Closed fracture of the pelvis is often the result of direct compression from heavy impact that crushes the bones. The force of energy can be a fall from a height or direct impact to the pelvis. Indirect force can also cause injury. For instance, when the knee strikes the dashboard, the force is transmitted along the femur, driving the femoral head into the pelvis, causing it to fracture. Not all fractures are from violent trauma; a simple fall can cause a closed fracture, especially in older adults.

A great deal of blood loss may occur from the large vessels in the retroperitoneal space adjacent to the pelvis. These vessels are easily torn or lacerated, with the blood draining into the retroperitoneal space. Most pelvic fractures are closed because heavy muscles surround and protect the pelvis. Occasionally, pieces of the pelvis will lacerate the rectum, vagina, or bladder. The bladder may also rupture. The structures that the pelvis is designed to protect, the bladder, rectum, vagina, and blood vessels, are all susceptible to damage when the pelvic ring is fractured. It should be assumed that a patient with a pelvic fracture has associated abdominal injuries until cleared by the physician.

Vascular Structures

Any of the abdominal vascular structures are subject to blunt or penetrating injuries. Often, the identification of specific vascular damage is not made until the patient is in surgery to repair other damage. In a stable patient, diagnostic CT scan and arteriography are used to identify the extent of vascular injury.

When disrupted, the aorta, inferior vena cava, iliac arteries, and hepatic veins hemorrhage severely, and death can be rapid if the damage is not repaired immediately. Emergency department management of vascular injuries pertains to IV access and getting the patient to the operating room as soon as possible.

ASSESSMENT

As with any injured patient, the ABCs and initial stabilization are the first priority. If the patient is critically injured or unstable, the physician may elect to go directly to surgery for immediate stabilization and repair of injuries. If the patient is relatively stable, he is assessed quickly and efficiently, under controlled circumstances.

Physical Examination

The abdominal examination should be performed in a standardized sequence: inspection, auscultation, percussion, and palpation.

1. **INSPECT** for abrasions, contusion from restraints, lacerations, impaled foreign bodies, evisceration of bowel, and pregnancy.

    — Seat belt sign is associated with mesenteric, bowel, lumbar, and spine injuries. They occur mostly in children with lap belt and no shoulder restraint.

2. **AUSCULTATION** of the abdomen in a noisy emergency department can be difficult.

    — Intraperitoneal blood can produce gastric ileus and thus silent bowel sounds. Other injuries to adjacent structures also cause ileus, so hypoactive bowel sounds are not diagnostic for abdominal injury alone.

3. **PERCUSSION** may elicit subtle signs of peritonitis. Tympanic sounds may indicate gastric dilatation, whereas dullness indicates hemoperitoneum.

4. **PALPATION** can reveal rebound tenderness when the palpating hand compresses and is removed quickly from the abdomen.

    — The presence of a pregnant uterus, as well as estimation of fetal age, also can be determined.

- Serial examinations by the same clinician improves sensitivity.

- Spinal cord injury masks clinical findings.

- Kehr's sign is left shoulder pain associated with hemoperitoneum and spleen injuries.

Perineal and Rectal Examination

Presence of blood at the urethral meatus strongly suggests a urethral tear. Rectal examination reveals valuable information. In blunt trauma, it is used to assess sphincter tone, position of the prostate, and to determine the presence of pelvic fractures. In penetrating trauma, gross blood indicates bowel perforation.

Vaginal Examination

Inspect and palpate for lacerations of the vagina, which can occur from bony fragments from pelvic fractures.

TUBES

Gastric Tube

Gastric tube placement decompresses the stomach to reduce the chance of aspiration. It should also be inserted prior to performing a diagnostic peritoneal lavage, to reduce the chance of perforating a distended stomach. Blood in the gastric aspirate suggests an injury to the esophagus or upper GI tract. Use caution when inserting a nasogastric tube if facial fractures or basilar skull fracture exist. Orogastric tubes are preferred in these situations to prevent passage of the tube into the brain.

Urinary Catheter

A Foley catheter is inserted to monitor urine output and to relieve retention and decompress the bladder prior to diagnostic peritoneal lavage. Hematuria is a possible sign of trauma to the genitourinary tract.

LABORATORY TESTS

- Baseline hematocrit

- Baseline creatinine

  — Prior to abdominal CT or angiography with contrast, check the baseline kidney function.

- Urinalysis

  — Absence of hematuria does not rule out genitourinary injury.

  — Presence of hematuria mandates consideration of a genitourinary injury.

- Elevated amylase/lipase or liver enzymes increasing the suspicion for intrabdominal injury

- Pregnancy test in women of childbearing age

DIAGNOSTIC TESTS

Table 8-3 lists the diagnostic tests that are useful for the identification of abdominal trauma.

ASSESSMENT PRINCIPLES

- If a patient is in shock with a penetrating injury or has a distended abdomen, it should be assumed that he has a major vascular injury until proven otherwise.

TABLE 8-3: DIAGNOSTIC TESTS FOR ABDOMINAL TRAUMA	
Flat Plate Abdominal X-ray	• Useful to detect free air under the diaphragm from a ruptured hollow viscus (organ) which mandates prompt operation • Useful to detect presence of bullets to estimate trajectory
Abdominal Ultrasound or Focused Assessment Sonography in Trauma (FAST)	• Useful in hemodynamically unstable patients • Quickly detects the presence of abdominal blood in unstable patients • Requires specific equipment in experienced hands • Is rapid, noninvasive, inexpensive • Should be repeated more then once to detect slow bleeding
Diagnostic Peritoneal Lavage (DPL)	• Not commonly used anymore; increasingly replaced by abdominal ultrasound (FAST) • Rapidly performed invasive procedure • To be performed by surgical team who will operate • Highly sensitive to detect intraperitoneal bleeding • Not useful to identify specific injuries • Does not diagnose retroperitoneal injuries
CT Scan	• Abdominal scanning for <u>specific</u> organ injury • Used in hemodynamically stable patients • Useful to identify retroperitoneal injuries
Urethrogram	• Used to detect injury of the urethra
Cystogram	• Used to detect a bladder injury
Intravenous Pyelogram (IVP)	• Used to detect ureter or kidney injury
Arteriography	• Used to detect vascular bleeding of abdominal and genitourinary organs

- If it is suspected that the patient has abdominal vascular injury, massive transfusions should be anticipated, including the replacement of platelets and plasma.

- Note how the patient is positioned. Pain may cause guarding in an attempt to protect the injured area. The patient may have difficulty moving or have his or her knees drawn up to his or her chest to relieve pressure and make it easier to breathe. He or she may be taking rapid, shallow breaths to minimize abdominal movement.

- Pain is a significant finding and its cause actively pursued.

- Nausea is a likely symptom with abdominal trauma.

- Vomiting may occur with the nausea.

- Tenderness, particularly if localized, is a significant sign indicating there may be internal damage.

- If the patient is developing peritonitis, he or she will want to lie still because any movement is painful.

- Abdominal distention or rigidity is an indicator of hemorrhage.

- Bruising and discoloration around the umbilicus is called Cullen's sign, which may indicate intraperitoneal hemorrhage.

- Bruising of the flank is Grey Turner's sign, and is associated with bleeding into the abdominal wall.

- Other signs of hemorrhage are hypotension, tachycardia, and pallor; hematemesis; hematuria, or blood (prostate disruption) at the meatus; and inability to urinate.

- Obvious deformity of the abdomen, evisceration of abdominal contents, or impalement may be associated with multiple abdominal injuries.

- Penetrating injuries cause wounds that are obvious on inspection, which make it somewhat easier to predict the extent of the injuries. Look for both entry and exit wounds.

- High velocity missiles often leave a small, harmless-looking wound at the entry point and a huge, gaping wound at the exit point. Always turn the patient over and examine him or her thoroughly for a possible exit wound.

- Bruising and swelling diagonally across the chest and/or abdomen indicates seat belt injury from deceleration.

MANAGEMENT AND INTERVENTION

- As with any injury, the first priorities are the ABCs and maintaining the airway.

- Serial vital signs, with temperature, should be monitored and recorded frequently, and any changes should be promptly reported to the physician. Look for signs of shock.

- Delayed diagnosis and treatment is a major cause of death.

- Because of the possibility of hemorrhage, two IV lines should be started immediately with large-bore needles.

- Be alert to indicators of multiple trauma and spinal injury. Abdominal trauma usually involves damage of more than one structure or organ. Look and feel for obvious deformities, tenderness, or abdominal tension.

- Ask the patient to describe the location and kind of pain he or she is feeling. Identify if the pain is direct and/or referred.

- Avoid excessive administration of pain medication until the physician has examined the patient. Other means of pain relief, such as position, reassurance, mouth care, and breathing techniques will help. The patient will be anxious and fearful.

- Observe for signs and symptoms of internal hemorrhaging: hypovolemic shock, abdominal pain and distention, and enlarging abdomen.

- If there is any indication of a fractured pelvis,

immobilize the patient. There may be a urethral or bladder disruption.

- Insert a Foley catheter only after a rectal examination has been performed by the physician so that a urethral injury is first ruled out.

- Anticipate blood administration in unstable abdominal trauma. Blood should be typed and crossmatched for at least 4 units or according to hospital policy.

- Do not remove an impaled object, as it is likely to tamponade the bleeding. Stabilize the object, and reassure the patient as to why this is being done. The object will be removed in a surgical environment where repairs can be made.

- Any body parts that are protruding from a wound should not be returned to the abdominal cavity. Cover with a sterile dressing moistened with normal saline solution.

- The patient cannot drink or eat anything until he or she is cleared regarding surgical intervention and has no evidence of nausea or vomiting.

- The patient should be kept warm. He or she is likely to be hypothermic, which increases the need for oxygen, decreases perfusion, causes coagulation problems, and decreases the chances of successful resuscitation. Warming the fluids and humidifying the oxygen reduces heat loss, as do head wraps and warming blankets.

- Be sure to explain to the patient the purpose for multiple tests and procedures if injuries are not evident; reassure him or her that tests are for thorough diagnosis and evaluation purposes.

DEFINITIVE TREATMENT

The nurse should anticipate the physician's orders. Be prepared to assist the patient for FAST, abdominal CT, angiography, or surgery. Admission to critical care for nonoperative management is also growing in popularity.

SUMMARY

Abdominal injuries present many assessment challenges and represent 25% of all traumatic injuries. The extent of an abdominal injury is probably one of the most frequently missed diagnoses, and if unrecognized, is one of the major causes of death from trauma.

EXAM QUESTIONS

CHAPTER 8

Questions 50-55

50. When a patient with reported abdominal injuries arrives in the emergency department, the sequence of physical examination of the abdomen is

    a. auscultate, inspect, percuss, palpate.

    b. percuss, auscultate, inspect, palpate.

    c. inspect, auscultate, percuss, palpate.

    d. palpate, inspect, auscultate, percuss.

51. Which of the following is true about blunt genitourinary trauma?

    a. Genitourinary organs are unprotected.

    b. Genitourinary injuries occur in isolation.

    c. Both kidneys are usually injured together.

    d. The urinary bladder is more likely to rupture when it is full.

52. The organ most likely to be damaged from blunt abdominal trauma is the

    a. liver.

    b. pancreas.

    c. spleen.

    d. small bowel.

53. The organ injuries that can be expected to bleed the most are

    a. kidney, spleen, liver.

    b. ureter, urethra, bladder.

    c. stomach, duodenum, colon.

    d. gallbladder, cecum, rectum.

54. A passenger in a motorcycle accident is brought to the emergency department with the history of being struck broadside at a speed of 50 mph. The patient cannot move her hips or legs without severe pain; she is bleeding from the vagina and rectum. Likely diagnosis is

    a. fractured patella and contusion to the abdomen.

    b. multiple contusions to the lower extremities.

    c. fractured pelvis, laceration of the rectum and vagina.

    d. fracture of the head of the femur, with abdominal contusions.

55. A 17-year-old female is struck by a truck traveling 50 mph. She has obvious fractures of the right tibia and fibula, pain in the pelvic area, and severe dyspnea. Her heart rate is 170 beats/min, and her respiratory rate is 46 breaths/min with no breath sounds heard in the left chest. A tension pneumothorax is relieved by immediate needle decompression and tube thoracostomy. Subsequently, her heart rate decreased to 140 beats/min, her respiratory rate decreases to 36 breaths/min, and her blood pressure is 80/50 mm Hg. Warmed lactated Ringer's solution is administered IV. In order to quickly identify the source of bleeding, the next intervention would be to

    a. perform external fixation of the pelvis.

    b. obtain abdominal and pelvic CT scans.

    c. perform a cystogram and urethrogram.

    d. perform an abdominal ultrasound (FAST).

CHAPTER 9

SPINAL TRAUMA

CHAPTER OBJECTIVE

Upon completion of this chapter, the reader will be able to relate the proper procedures for managing spinal injuries.

LEARNING OBJECTIVES

Upon completion of this chapter, the reader should be able to

1. identify basic spinal anatomy and physiology.

2. identify common characteristics of spinal cord injury.

3. recognize a patient with suspected spinal cord injury.

4. recognize frequently seen spinal cord injuries.

5. choose assessment priorities for the trauma patient with an injured spinal cord.

INTRODUCTION

Spinal cord injuries are often catastrophic as nearly half of the injuries involve the cervical spine, and nearly half of that result in quadriplegia. The financial cost alone to society is estimated to be billions of dollars annually (McQuillan et al., 2002).

The most common cause of spinal injury is the motor vehicle crash (MVC): head-on collisions, rollovers, ejection, and collisions with pedestrians. These injuries make up at least half of the acute cases. Falls, direct blows to the head or neck, sports injuries (such as football and diving), and penetrating wounds from guns or knives make up a large portion of the rest of the injuries. As recreational and technological opportunities expand, the means for spinal cord injury increase. In recent years, in-line skating, extreme skiing, snowboarding, and cycling have added to the mechanisms of injury. Upper cervical injury is increasingly identified as a cause of death in cases of child abuse, particularly infants. "Shaken baby" trauma causes acceleration-deceleration damage to the brain. Because the infant's head is relatively large and heavy and the neck is weak, the brain bounces back and forth in the cranium, causing eventual tearing of the cortical veins, along with cervical injury.

Since the development of emergency medical services (EMS) as a system in the early 1970s along with advanced prehospital and emergency department care, more people sustaining spinal cord injuries survive, and many survive in better condition. The rapid advanced medical interventions along with spinal cord rehabilitation systems across the country have decreased complications and brought about better recovery potential for those injured. However, because more survive, more people are left with seriously debilitating and crippling injuries. Today, society has become more knowledgeable and accepting about adapting to, and including, those with spinal cord injuries in the workforce, sports, and the social world.

ANATOMY AND PHYSIOLOGY

Overview

A "system" is a combination of interrelated parts forming a complex or unitary whole. The body's nervous system is a perfect example of a complex unitary whole having several components or interrelated systems. It literally controls all activities of the body.

Anatomical

Anatomically, the nervous system has two divisions: the **central nervous system** (CNS) and the **peripheral nervous system** (PNS) (see Figure 9-1).

The CNS consists of the brain and spinal cord. The brain is the controlling organ of the body, serving as the center of consciousness, directing voluntary and involuntary activities, perceiving one's surroundings, and controlling reactions to those surroundings. It receives and sorts information and directs the body's response. It is the brain that enables us to experience thought and feelings. Three major subdivisions of the brain are the cerebrum, cerebellum, and brain stem. The brain stem is the continuous portion of the brain that joins with the spinal cord and functions as an important relay and reflex center. It is the most primitive part of the CNS, and controls all the body functions necessary for life.

The spinal cord is the part of the CNS that transmits messages back and forth between the brain and the body. As in the brain, the spinal cord has cell bodies, but it is mostly made up of nerve fibers extending from the brain to just below the brain stem where it forms the spinal cord. Many nerve cells in the CNS have long fibers that continue outside the system to form cables of nerve fibers linking the CNS to various organs in the body.

The linking cables of nerve fibers reaching outside the CNS make up the PNS. This system includes the nerves that enter and leave the spinal cord and those that connect the brain and organs

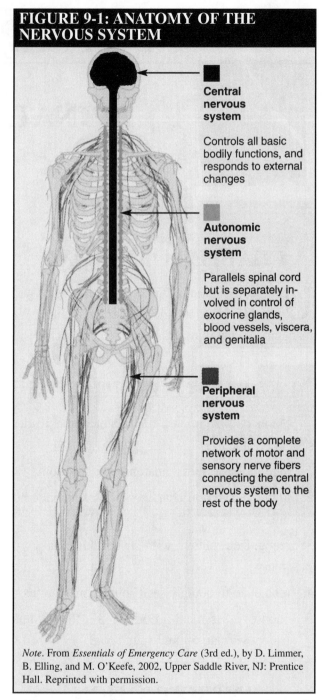

FIGURE 9-1: ANATOMY OF THE NERVOUS SYSTEM

Central nervous system

Controls all basic bodily functions, and responds to external changes

Autonomic nervous system

Parallels spinal cord but is separately involved in control of exocrine glands, blood vessels, viscera, and genitalia

Peripheral nervous system

Provides a complete network of motor and sensory nerve fibers connecting the central nervous system to the rest of the body

Note. From *Essentials of Emergency Care* (3rd ed.), by D. Limmer, B. Elling, and M. O'Keefe, 2002, Upper Saddle River, NJ: Prentice Hall. Reprinted with permission.

without passing through the cord, such as the optic nerve. There are 31 pairs of peripheral nerves, called spinal nerves, and 12 pairs of cranial nerves.

The cranial nerves arise from the brain stem, each having a name and corresponding Roman numeral, and pass directly through holes in the skull to their innervations. They may be sensory nerves, motor nerves, or both. Mostly, cranial nerves are specialized and have particular functions in the head and face.

The 31 pairs of spinal nerves provide pathways for responses to specific stimuli. Each nerve has paired roots that extend from either side of the spinal cord to transmit sensory and motor impulses. The paired nerves correspond to specific segments of the spinal cord and are: 8 cervical, 12 thoracic, 5 lumbar, 5 sacral, and 1 coccygeal nerve.

Three categories of peripheral nerves are sensory, motor, and connecting nerves. Sensory nerves carry messages sent from the body to the central nervous system. Sensory nerves are complex and are made up of many types of cells, such as those in the retina, ear, skin, muscles, joints, and organs. They do as the name implies and detect sensations of heat, cold, position, motion, pressure, light, hearing, balance, taste, smell, and many others. Each cell has distinctive nerve endings that only perceive one type of sensation and send only one type of message. Cranial sensory nerves go directly to the brain and do not pass through the spinal cord.

The nerves sending messages from the CNS to the muscles are motor nerves. Each muscle in the body has its own motor nerve. An impulse in the motor strip of the brain's cerebral cortex is sent along the spinal cord to a cell body. The receiving cell body in the spinal cord then transmits the impulse to the motor nerve of the specific muscle it causes to contract.

In the brain and spinal cord are cells, the connecting nerves, with short fibers that connect the sensory nerves with the motor nerves. Some connect directly in the spinal cord without having to go through the brain, allowing the nerves to transmit impulses between nerves within the CNS. Connecting nerves in the spinal cord form a reflex arc between sensory and motor nerves of the extremities. When an irritating stimulus is transmitted from the sensory nerve along the connecting nerve directly to the motor nerve, immediate response occurs, even before the information can be sent to the brain. Examples of reflex reactions are the responses that occur when one touches some-thing extremely hot or when the physician taps the patellar tendon.

Functional

Aside from the anatomical divisions of the nervous system, there are functional divisions: the somatic and autonomic nervous systems.

Activities that are voluntary and which one has control over, such as walking and writing, are controlled by the **somatic nervous system.** The peripheral nerves send sensory information to the brain for interpretation. The brain then responds to the voluntary muscles to act.

In the involuntary or **autonomic nervous system,** one has no conscious or deliberate control over the functions it governs such as digestion, dilation and constriction of blood vessels, and perspiring.

Some of the cells forming the autonomic system are inside the CNS and others lie alongside the spinal cord near the point where the spinal nerve roots exit. There are two branches of the autonomic system: the sympathetic and the parasympathetic.

Along the vertebral column, a chain of ganglia (a collection of nerve-cell bodies) form the main sympathetic trunks that extend from the base of the skull to the coccyx. They are supplied by the thoracolumbar portion of the spinal cord nerve roots. The **sympathetic system** responds to stress and threatening situations by causing the pupils to dilate, blood vessels to constrict, stimulating sweating, increasing the heart rate, causing sphincter muscles to constrict, and preparing the body to respond to stress.

The **parasympathetic system** is the other side of the sympathetic coin, the balancing side. The parasympathetic nerve cells are found in the brain stem and the sacral area of the spinal cord. They cause the pupils to constrict, blood vessels to dilate, slow the heart rate, and relax the sphincters and other responses.

Autonomic functions include slowing or increasing the heart rate and strength of contractions, dilating or constricting blood vessels in skeletal muscles and abdominal organs, changing bronchial diameter, relaxing or contracting the urinary bladder, dilating or constricting the pupils, and increasing or decreasing saliva and digestive juices. Any injury interfering with the function of the autonomic system can be life threatening.

To summarize, the nervous system is anatomically divided into the CNS and the PNS. Functionally, the nervous system is made up of the somatic and autonomic components.

The Spinal Cord

The purpose of the spinal cord is to transmit nerve messages, or impulses, back and forth between the brain and the body in order to control functions and movements. Impulses are electrical, moving along nerve fibers within the spinal cord.

Nerve fibers in the spinal cord are grouped together in tracts. Sensory input from the body to the spinal cord is received by the ascending tracts and brain commands for body motor functions travel through the descending tracts. While it is not necessary to know the names of all the tracts, it is important to know that the functions of three tracts relate to position sense, pain sense, and movement, and should be assessed after an injury.

The base of the skull has an opening, the foramen magnum, through which the spinal cord exits to enter the spinal canal down to the lumbar vertebrae. Meninges covering the brain continue down to surround the cord, which is about 2.5 in. (1 cm) in diameter. Fluid that bathes and cushions the brain also surrounds the cord, which is why it is called cerebrospinal fluid (CSF).

The spinal cord is housed in the spinal column (see Figure 9-2). It is well protected by 33 vertebrae, aligned by strong ligaments that connect, support, provide stability, and prevent excessive flexion or extension of the vertebrae. The vertebrae support the head and body, allowing a person to walk upright. Segments of the vertebrae are: 7 cervical,

FIGURE 9-2: ANATOMY OF THE SPINE

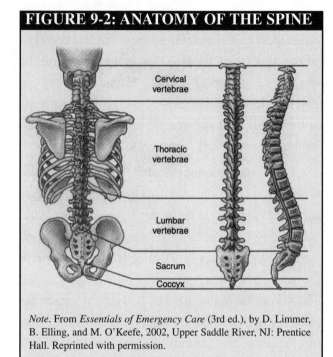

Note. From *Essentials of Emergency Care* (3rd ed.), by D. Limmer, B. Elling, and M. O'Keefe, 2002, Upper Saddle River, NJ: Prentice Hall. Reprinted with permission.

12 thoracic, 5 lumbar, 5 fused sacral, and 4 fused coccygeal.

Between each of the cervical, thoracic, and lumbar vertebrae are broad, flat, intervertebral discs made of fibrocartilage. They act as shock absorbers for the vertebrae. The vascular supply is the vertebral artery and spinal rami arteries entering between the vertebrae. Different from other areas of the body, spinal arteries cannot develop an adequate collateral blood supply when they are injured or obstructed.

Mechanism of Injury

Adult Patients

The major causes of adult spinal trauma include car crashes, shallow water diving/swimming, motorcycle crashes, and all other falls and injuries. Rapid forward deceleration during an MVC and rapid vertical deceleration from a fall are the two primary causes of injury to the spine. Patients over age 45 have more spinal injuries from falls than MVCs (see Figure 9-3).

Pediatric Patients

Pediatric patient frequency and injury patterns are quite different. Most pediatric spinal injuries are

FIGURE 9-3: MECHANISMS OF BLUNT SPINAL INJURY

DESCRIPTION	DIAGRAM	EXAMPLES
Hyperextension Excessive posterior movement of head or neck	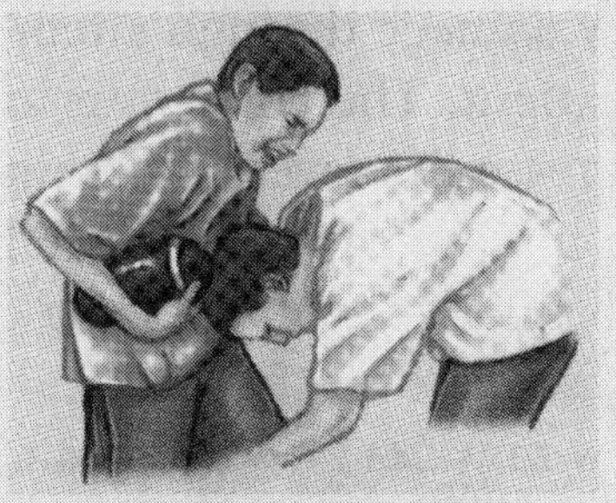	Face into windshield in motor vehicle crash (MVC) Elderly person falling to the floor Football tackler Dive into shallow water
Hyperflexion Excessive anterior movement of head onto chest	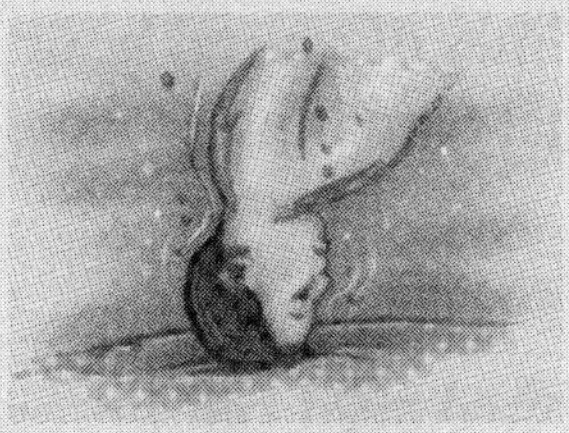	Rider thrown off horse or motorcycle Dive into shallow water
Compression Weight of head or pelvis driven into stationary neck or torso	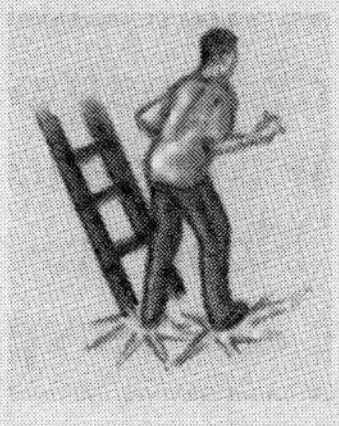	Dive into shallow water Fall of greater than 10 to 20 feet onto head or legs
Rotation Excessive rotation of the torso or head and neck, moving one side of the spinal column against the other	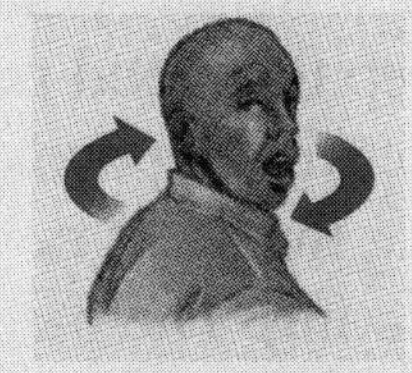	Rollover MVC Motorcycle accident
Lateral Stress Direct lateral force on spinal column, typically shearing one level of cord from another	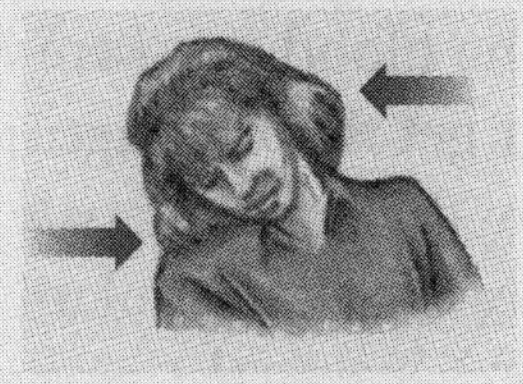	"T-bone" MVC Fall
Distraction Excessive stretching of column and cord	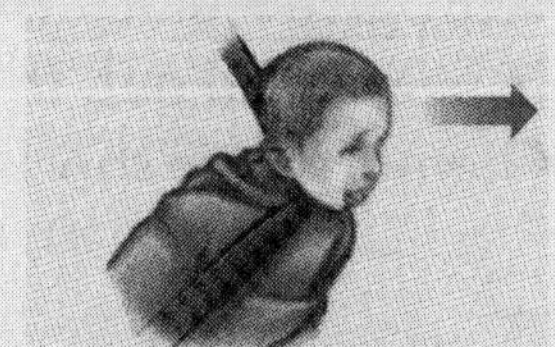	Hanging Child inappropriately wearing shoulder belt around neck Snowmobile or motorcycle under rope or wire

Note. From *Basic Trauma Life Support for Advanced Providers*, by J. Campbell, Ed., 2004, Upper Saddle River, NJ: Prentice Hall. Reprinted with permission.

the result of falling, either from a height or bicycle; being struck by a car; diving accidents; or sports-related injuries.

Injury can occur to the spinal cord, bony column, or both at the same time. Ligament sprains usually are uncomplicated and heal without problems. Trauma to the spinal column does not always affect the cord or the nerves. Not all vertebral injuries are fractures. Trauma to the spine severe enough to injure the cord is usually severe enough to make the spinal column unstable. The most common sites of injury are in descending order – cervical spine, followed by thoracic, thoracolumbar, and lumbarsacral.

Penetrating Injury

When projectiles or other penetrating forces enter the spinal cord, they can cause shearing. Structure and function can be disrupted or ended. Bone fragments may be driven into the spinal cord with penetrating force, causing further damage.

Bleeding or a hematoma at the trauma site can compress the spinal cord; and loss of blood supply can bring about irreversible damage. If damage is severe enough, the patient will have partial or complete loss of bodily sensation or function. Loss starts at the site of the injury and continues downward. If the injury is high level and severe in the cervical cord, it is life-threatening due to loss of the ability of the respiratory system to function on its own.

Neurogenic Shock

Neurogenic shock results from impairment of the descending sympathetic pathways in the spinal cord. There is a loss of vasomotor tone, which results in vasodilatation and hypotension. There is also a loss of sympathetic innervation of the heart, which can result in bradycardia or at least a failure to become tachycardic in response to hypovolemia.

Spinal Shock

Spinal shock refers to flaccidity and the temporary loss of reflexes seen after spinal cord injury. The "shock" to the cord makes it appear impaired but not necessarily destroyed. The duration of the loss of reflexes is variable.

Spinal Cord Injury Classified by Level

Cervical Spine Injury (C1-C7)

The most common cervical injury is fracture or subluxation of C5. The diaphragm is innervated by the phrenic nerve between C3 and C5. Therefore, trauma to the upper-or middle-cervical cord often paralyzes intercostal muscles resulting in hypoventilation or apnea. Many people with high-cervical spine injuries die at the scene of respiratory distress before assistance arrives.

- There is an association between cervical spine injuries and head injuries.
  - Approximately 5% of brain-injured patients have an associated spinal injury, while 25% of spinal injury patients have at least a mild brain injury. (American College of Surgeons, 2004b)
- Never assume there is only one fracture of the spine.
  - Approximately 10% of patients with a cervical spine fracture have a second bony column fracture elsewhere.
  - A high index of suspicion for a second spine injury is necessary to avoid a missed injury.
- Remember the patient will have inability to perceive pain, which can mask a potentially serious injury elsewhere, such as the abdomen.

Thoracic Spine Injury (T1-T10)

The thoracic spine receives additional stability from the ribs. Therefore, it is not injured as often as other parts of the spine. However, when a fracture-dislocation in the thoracic spine does occur, it almost always results in a complete neurologic deficit because of the relatively narrow dimension of the thoracic canal. If thoracic injury is suspected, the neck must also be stabilized.

- **Compression fractures** are common in the thoracic region and are usually stable.

- **Burst fractures** caused by vertical-axial compression is also common. These are unstable and require surgery.

- **Chance fractures** are transverse fractures through the vertebral body and are most commonly seen following MVCs in which the patient (usually a child) was restrained only by a lap belt.

Thoracolumbar Injury

The lumbar and thoracic vertebrae join as a flexible joint, which makes it subject to injury. The T-12 to L-1 area is the second most common site for injury in the spine (American College of Surgeons, 2004b). Spinal cord damage to the lumbar region can paralyze the legs.

Spinal Cord Syndromes

Complete Cord Transection

A complete spinal cord injury is when there is no demonstrable sensory or motor function below a certain level. The diagnosis cannot be made for the first few days after injury until spinal shock is ruled out.

Anterior Cord Syndrome

Anterior cord syndrome is characterized by paraplegia and sensory loss with loss of pain and temperature. With the posterior part of the spinal column still intact, the patient is able to feel vibrations and has proprioception. Usually, anterior cord syndrome is caused by infarction of the cord in the territory supplied by the anterior spinal artery. This syndrome has a poor prognosis.

Central Cord Syndrome

Central cord syndrome is caused most often by hyperextension, especially by older people in a fall in which they strike their face. Loss of function is in the upper extremities but not in the lower extremities. Prognosis for recovery is good.

Brown-Séquard Syndrome

Brown-Séquard syndrome is cord damage limited to one hemisphere. It is rarely seen and usually results from penetrating trauma. Characteristics of this syndrome are ipsilateral (same side) motor loss and proprioception along with contralateral loss of pain and temperature sensation. Prognosis is fair with some recovery usually seen.

Penetrating Injury

The nature of penetrating injury is that there are open wounds into the spinal cord. If CSF is evident, the spinal cord has been perforated, and infection is likely along with the injury.

Injury Without Radiographic Abnormality

A child's anatomy allows for more physical flexibility than that of an adult. As a result, spinal cord injury is less likely. However, a condition known as spinal cord injury without radiographic abnormality (SCIWORA) can occur, where the child shows signs of injury without radiographic evidence. It is thought that a young child's immaturely developed spinal column can accept more flexion and extension without demonstrable vertebral damage. Consequently, when damage occurs, it may not be immediately obvious but may progress over hours or days. The injury is more likely to occur at the cervical or thoracic levels of the spinal cord and show neurologic deficits without evidence of bony injury. A magnetic resonance imaging (MRI) is required to detect the specific point of injury.

Initial Assessment

The emergency nurse should first conduct primary and secondary assessments and initiate critical interventions that are required. All patients who are unconscious should be presumed to have multisystem injury or spinal injury. They should arrive at the emergency department fully immobilized on a backboard and kept that way until cleared by the physician. The patient should have a hard cervical collar and lateral head support. Remember not to rely exclusively on the collar, as it does not fully immobilize the patient. Once the patient's critical needs have been met, a more focused assessment related to the spinal injury can be conducted.

Signs

Unconsciousness: The accepted rule is that an unconscious patient is assumed to have a spinal injury until proven otherwise and cleared by the physician.

Deformity: Although deformity is an obvious indicator of injury, most spinal cord and spinal fractures do not have obvious deformity. Only when there is severe injury with marked displacement of bony fragments is deformity obvious. Absence of deformity does not indicate lack of a fracture or displacement. When present, a deformity is most often seen in the cervical spine with the head twisted to one side.

Tenderness: Point tenderness over any part of the spine indicates injury. The spinous processes of all the cervical, thoracic, and lumbar vertebrae can (are able to) be palpated; with C7 being especially prominent.

Lacerations or contusions: Cuts and bruises often occur with strong force. A cervical spine injury usually results from a blow to the head. If the head or face is marked with lacerations or contusions, it is a reliable indication that there may be spinal injury. Patients with serious lacerations or contusions over areas of the back, shoulders, or abdomen are likely to have injuries to the spine.

Paralysis: Weakness or loss of sensation identified during assessment by touching the fingers, toes, arms, and legs is a sign of spinal injury. Upper extremity muscle strength is tested by judging the grip when the patient is asked to squeeze the nurse's hand. Lower extremity muscle strength is tested by asking the patient to move his or her feet up and down.

Respiratory Difficulty: Difficulty breathing or inability to breathe may indicate cervical or thoracic damage.

Priapism: Priapism indicates loss of sympathetic nervous system control and parasympathetic stimulation.

Symptoms

Pain: Pain due to spinal injury is an important indicator. The nurse should document where the pain is, the quality of pain, and if it increases with movement, should the patient try to move. The nurse should not ask the patient to move.

Numbness or Tingling: Damage to the spine probably has occurred if the patient complains of numbness, tingling, loss of feeling, or weakness.

History

If the patient is conscious when he arrives at the emergency department, it is important to verify the mechanism of injury and history that has been recorded by the rescue crew. With a suspected spine injury, signs and symptoms should be evaluated for any changes or increase in complaints. If the patient is unconscious, prehospital history is what the nurse has to rely on, along with report from the rescuers.

Information should include:

- History of significant trauma, such as a motor vehicle or motorcycle crash or a fall from a height greater than three times the patient's height, especially if there is a fracture of the heels

- Unrestrained driver or passenger

- Facial trauma

- Loss of consciousness at the site of the injury

- Altered mental status from intoxication or drugs

- Any seizure activity since the injury

- Neck pain or altered sensation in the upper extremities

- Neck tenderness

- Injury above the clavicle

- Chest or intra-abdominal injuries

- Confirm if the patient has been incontinent before arrival at the emergency department or, if a male, is experiencing priapism

Assessment

- Look for obvious signs of injury.

- Look for abnormal shape of the spine and cervical edema.

- Identify the patient's breathing pattern, and document difficulties.

- Injury above C-6 disrupts ventilation. Abdominal breathing can indicate damage from C-3 to C-5.

- Document if the patient can move extremities and perceive pain.

- Priapism is associated with loss of sympathetic system control, indicated in cervical injury.

- Feel the patient's skin. If it is cool and looks pink, the patient may have neurogenic shock.

- Perform a quick motor evaluation, assessing the strength and equality of movement for all four extremities, including the feet, toes, hands, and fingers.

- Briefly assess sensory status to identify if the patient can distinguish between sharp and dull and identify where there is loss of feeling.

Management of Spinal Cord and Column Injuries

The purpose of spinal cord trauma management is the same as with any fracture: support and immobilize. The principle of immobilization is in-line position and immobilization of the joint above and below the fracture. For immobilization of any spinal injury, the anatomy of the spine dictates that the joint above refers to the head and the joint below refers to the torso and pelvis.

Because the extent of spinal injuries cannot be completely observed and because they may become progressively worse, spinal injuries should always be considered serious and potentially totally disabling or life-threatening.

Unfortunately, at least 5% of patients experience worsening of preexisting neurologic deficit after reaching the emergency department. This is usually due to ischemia or progression of spinal cord edema, but it may also be due to inadequate spinal immobilization. (American College of Surgeons, 2004b).

Stabilization

- Spine trauma patient stabilization begins with identification and treatment of airway and vascular compromise. While the ABCs are conducted, the cervical spine must be well immobilized, as is necessary if an airway has to be established and ventilation maintained.

- The only acceptable method to open the airway of a patient with a cervical injury is the jaw thrust maneuver.

- Cervical spine trauma puts the patient at risk for hypoxia, respiratory arrest, and aspiration.

- The airway is at risk for several problems: compromised respiratory muscles, localized edema causing obstruction of the airway, and penetration of the airway.

- Advanced airway measures may have to be taken, requiring special care to immobilize the neck.

- If the patient does not have a facial or cranial injury, the airway of choice is nasal intubation because it can be done with minimal spine manipulation.

- Administer oxygen to all patients with a suspected or known spinal injury to increase the oxygen supply to the spinal cord.

Immobilization

The nurse must ensure the patient is correctly immobilized:

- If the patient should arrive without immobilization, a rigid collar must be immediately applied.

Use a rigid cervical collar, lateral head immobilizer, and backboard. The size must be correct; a collar that is too large will cause hyperextension. Someone should help apply the collar to ensure in-line stabilization of the spine.

- Care should be taken that the collar does not block the mouth.

- Do not overly rely on cervical collars; they do not hold the head absolutely still and permit some side-to-side movement.

- In the concern for the spine injury immobilization, be sure that other injuries are not aggravated when immobilizing devices are applied.

- Do not remove a helmet unless it is essential for accessing the airway, sustaining respirations, or controlling hemorrhage.

Spinal Board Immobilization

Prehospital care personnel usually immobilize patients on long spine boards prior to their transport to the emergency department. Once the patient arrives at the emergency department however, every effort should be made to get the patient off the spine board as early as possible to reduce the risk of decubitus ulcer formation. Removal of the board is often done as part of the secondary survey when the patient is log rolled for inspection and palpation of the back. Some trauma centers remove the board within 20 min of arrival. Boards should never be used for longer than 2 hr for risk of skin breakdown. The cervical collar should be left on and the patient log rolled when moved to and from examination or operating room tables. The patient can be placed back on the board if and when transfer to another facility is required.

Circulation

Neurogenic shock will cause hypotension, flushed skin, and bradycardia. If hypotension occurs, carefully verify that it is not caused by another problem, such as hypovolemia, tension pneumothorax, or intra-abdominal bleeding.

Patients with no obvious signs of bleeding who remain hypotensive should raise the suspicion of neurogenic shock. If blood pressure does not improve after fluid challenge, then judicious use of vasopressors may be warranted.

Excessive fluid administration can cause pulmonary edema. Invasive monitoring such as central venous pressure monitoring may be helpful in guiding fluid administration. If the patient has spinal cord damage, he may not be able to feel the sensation of a full bladder. After it is confirmed there is no urethral damage, Foley catheterization is usually necessary.

Pharmacological Management

If the patient arrives at the emergency department within 8 hr of the injury, high-dose methylprednisolone is usually administered to patients with nonpenetrating spinal cord injury. Although this is considered the current standard of care, recent research indicates high doses may put the patient at greater risk for pneumonia, decubitus ulcer development, and urinary tract infections. There is also a question as to whether early administration actually improves the functional status (American College of Surgeons, 2004a).

Transfer

Patients with spinal fractures and/or spinal cord injuries should be transferred to definitive care facilities. Avoid unnecessary delay. The spine should be stabilized prior to transfer with necessary splints, backboard, and semi-rigid cervical collar. Use caution with a patient with cervical injuries above C-6 due to potential respiratory embarrassment. If there is any concern about the airway, it is recommended that you intubate the patient prior to transfer.

SUMMARY

Spinal cord and spinal column injury can be devastating. The advancement of EMS systems and rehabilitation have improved the patient's chances of survival and expanded the potential for recovery. It is necessary to identify the cause and extent of an injury to the spinal cord or spine. Additionally, the patient must be carefully immobilized in order to prevent further damage. The future of the patient's ability to recover in the best manner possible depends upon prehospital and hospital staff who understand the principles of spinal cord and column injury and can appropriately manage the care of the patient.

EXAM QUESTIONS

CHAPTER 9

Questions 56-60

56. All messages that the brain sends for the body to function are sent through the

    a. vertebral ganglia.

    b. sensory and functional nervous systems.

    c. spinal cord.

    d. sympathetic and parasympathetic nervous systems.

57. Which of the following statements is true?

    a. Injury to the spinal cord always includes paralysis.

    b. Complete spinal cord trauma causes paralysis above the point of injury.

    c. Injury can occur to the spinal cord, bony column, or both at the same time.

    d. The slight displacement of a fractured vertebra will not damage the spinal cord.

58. The pathophysiology of neurogenic shock is primarily related to

    a. loss of deep tendon reflexes.

    b. decreased cardiac contractility.

    c. tachycardia.

    d. loss of vasomotor tone.

59. A 7-year-old boy is a back-seat restrained passenger in a car hit from behind at high speed. His blood pressure is 80/60 mm Hg, heart rate is 84 beats/min, and respiratory rate is 18 breaths/min. The GCS score is 14, and he complains that his legs "feel funny and won't move." Spinal x-rays however do not show any abnormality. A spinal cord injury in this child

    a. may exist without any specific x-ray findings.

    b. can be ruled out by obtaining a computed tomography (CT) scan of the entire spine.

    c. is most likely central cord syndrome.

    d. is exacerbated by neurogenic shock.

60. A 30-year-old man presents to the emergency department after sustaining a 20 foot fall from scaffolding. He is unable to move his legs and has some limited movement of his arms. The lateral cervical spine xray shows a subluxation of C5 on C6. Vital signs are BP 110/60, P100, RR 10. The nurse should anticipate the following management priority

    a. immediate MRI.

    b. assist with ventilation.

    c. prepare for surgery.

    d. log roll of backboard.

CHAPTER 10

MUSCULOSKELETAL TRAUMA

CHAPTER OBJECTIVE

Upon completion of this chapter, the reader will be able to identify the proper procedures for managing musculoskeletal trauma.

LEARNING OBJECTIVES

Upon completion of this chapter, the reader should be able to

1. specify basic structures and functions of the musculoskeletal system.

2. identify common mechanisms of injury associated with musculoskeletal trauma.

3. recognize the pathophysiologic changes as a basis for signs and symptoms.

4. describe the nursing assessment of the patient with musculoskeletal injuries.

5. specify appropriate interventions for musculoskeletal injuries.

INTRODUCTION

More than half of all trauma-related hospital admissions are patients with some type of fracture, usually of the lower extremity. (Moore et al., 2004) Musculoskeletal injuries, including fractures, dislocations, and sprains are a significant group in the emergency department population. Most of the mechanisms of injury are motor vehicle crashes (MVCs), assaults, falls, sports injuries, and injuries that are work- or home-related.

Orthopedic injuries are a significant cause of short- and long-term disabilities. Although injuries usually are not critical unless accompanied by severe hemorrhage, such as traumatic amputations, they may be urgent because of potential arterial occlusion or neurovascular damage.

Quick and appropriate evaluation and intervention may prevent permanent disability.

ANATOMY AND PHYSIOLOGY

Musculoskeletal and related neurovascular structures are bones, joints, tendons, ligaments, muscles, blood vessels, and nerves.

Bones

Bones are the 206 skeletal structures that provide support, give solidity, strength, movement, and protection to the body and its organs (see Figure 10-1). They are also involved in blood cell formation and storing calcium. Bones are richly supplied by blood vessels, nerves, and lymphatic vessels for nourishment and self-repair.

Ligaments connect bones to other bones, and tendons connect muscle to bone.

FIGURE 10-1: THE HUMAN SKELETON

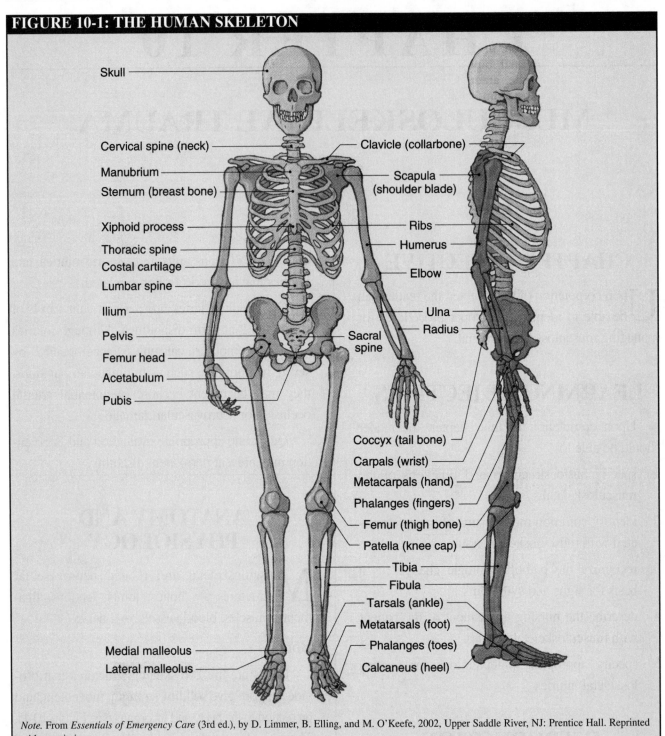

Skull
Cervical spine (neck)
Manubrium
Sternum (breast bone)
Xiphoid process
Thoracic spine
Costal cartilage
Lumbar spine
Ilium
Pelvis
Femur head
Acetabulum
Pubis
Medial malleolus
Lateral malleolus

Clavicle (collarbone)
Scapula (shoulder blade)
Ribs
Humerus
Elbow
Ulna
Radius
Sacral spine
Coccyx (tail bone)
Carpals (wrist)
Metacarpals (hand)
Phalanges (fingers)
Femur (thigh bone)
Patella (knee cap)
Tibia
Fibula
Tarsals (ankle)
Metatarsals (foot)
Phalanges (toes)
Calcaneus (heel)

Note. From *Essentials of Emergency Care* (3rd ed.), by D. Limmer, B. Elling, and M. O'Keefe, 2002, Upper Saddle River, NJ: Prentice Hall. Reprinted with permission.

Joints

A joint is the point of connection between two bones, held together by fibrous connective tissue and cartilage, the joint capsule. Functions of joints are to give stability and mobility, flexion and extension, medial and lateral rotation, and abduction and adduction. Movement is aided by muscles and ligaments connected with the joint.

Because of their function and location, joints are vulnerable to stress, inflammation, and trauma. Injuries occur in the form of contusions, sprains, dislocations, and penetration.

Muscle

Muscle facilitates movement. The body's 600 muscles basically are divided into three types: skeletal, smooth, and cardiac.

Skeletal or voluntary muscle forms the major muscle mass of the body and attaches to the skeletal bones. These muscles are under the direct control of the nervous system's commands to the brain, contracting or relaxing at will and related to all body movement. Specific nerves pass directly from the brain to the spinal cord, where they connect with other nerves leaving the spinal cord and then with each skeletal muscle.

Ligaments

Ligaments are sheets or bands of strong fibrous connective tissue that connect bone to bone at points of articulation. Their purpose is to align the bones and allow or limit motion.

Tendons

Cords of fibrous tissue that attach most skeletal muscle to bone are tendons. The cords are a continuation of the fascia covering all skeletal muscles, similar to the way skin covers a sausage. At each end of the muscle, the fascia continues beyond the muscle to attach to the bone, crossing the joint as the musculotendinous unit. It is this muscle-tendon unit that moves the joint.

Cartilage

Cartilage is a specialized type of dense connective tissue and has a limited vascular supply. It is found between the ribs, in the nasal septum, ear, larynx, trachea, bronchi, between the vertebrae, and articulating surfaces between bones.

MECHANISM OF INJURY

Blunt and penetrating, direct and indirect, twisting or high-energy trauma is involved in orthopedic and related neurovascular injuries. When there is trauma to the musculoskeletal system, dam-age also occurs to the surrounding tissues, such as the nerves and vessels. Musculoskeletal trauma can be sustained as a single system injury or in combination with other systems. Therefore, it is important not to focus on the assessment of a musculoskeletal injury to the exclusion of other possible injuries.

Considerable force is involved in fractures and dislocations. Twisting is often the cause of the tibial fractures and knee and ankle ligament injuries seen in athletic trauma. In cases of severe trauma, when the bones are broken and torn or sheared from the surrounding tissues, amputation occurs. Other times, when the bone does not break, tendons, ligaments, and muscles may be strained, sprained, or torn by the force of the trauma.

High-energy injury from auto crashes, falls from heights, gunshot wounds, or other extreme forces result in severe skeletal, surrounding soft tissue and adjacent vital organ damage. Multiple injuries generally are associated with high-energy trauma.

Penetrating injuries from gunshot wounds and knives may cause shattering of bones and lacerations of the muscles, tendons, and ligaments. When a projectile passes through bone, the bone fragments along with the foreign object cause additional tissue and structural damage. The ends of the broken bone may also protrude through the skin, inviting bacteria and infection along with bringing about additional tissue damage.

Age is a factor in the results of a musculoskeletal injury. With the same mechanism of injury, the older person may incur a fracture, while a younger person will have a dislocation. Twisting and rotational forces can fracture a bone along with rupturing ligaments and tendons and often are a hallmark of abuse in young children. Bicep tears may happen with relatively little effort in middle-aged or older adults.

ORTHOPEDIC TRAUMA AND ASSOCIATED NEUROVASCULAR PROBLEMS

Crush Injuries

Crush injuries range from the fingertip to a large body area. Mechanisms of injury are common in an industrial environment: conveyor belts, grinders, wringers, and machine presses, for example. Complications depend upon the specific mechanism of injury and the extent of damage. When there is tissue necrosis of a significant muscle mass, such as the thigh or calf, systemic crush syndrome causing rhabdomyolysis may occur. This is marked by extracellular fluid loss and myoglobinuria (myoglobin in the urine). Rhabdomyolysis may lead to hypovolemia, metabolic acidosis, hyperkalemia, hypocalcemia, and disseminated intravascular coagulation (DIC).

- The initiation of aggressive IV fluid therapy during resuscitation is critical to protecting the kidney and preventing renal failure.

- Osmotic diuresis and alkalization of the urine with sodium bicarbonate prevent precipitation of myoglobin in the tubules (American College of Surgeons, 2004a).

- Amputation of the crushed extremity may be necessary to prevent systemic complications as listed above.

Impaling Injuries

Impalements may occur secondary to falling on a piercing object, be sustained from machinery or pneumatic tools (nails from nail gun), or by an impaling object, either a weapon or other instrument. The wound will vary in size and the depth is difficult to determine. Sometimes, the object will still be embedded in the patient when he or she arrives at the emergency room.

- Impaled objects should not be removed.

- Secure the object with padding and dressings as much as possible.

- Surgical intervention may be necessary for removal of the object.

Dislocations

Defined as a complete loss of articular contact between two bones in a joint, dislocation causes direct injury to ligaments and capsule tissues. It is essential to assess the pulse carefully and serially.

- Palpate and splint the joint in the position as it presents and until the physician manages the injury.

- If reduction is necessary, it will be conducted with analgesia and sedation, and the patient is carefully monitored.

Shoulder Dislocation

Shoulder dislocation is probably the most commonly dislocated joint in children and athletes There are two areas affected:

Anterior

Anterior dislocations are generally seen in athletic injuries when there is a fall on an extended arm that is abducted and externally rotated. The force pushes the humeral head in front of the shoulder joint.

Posterior

Not frequently seen, posterior dislocations can occur in seizure patients when the arm is abducted and internally rotated. Place the patient in the position of most comfort.

- Evaluate distal pulses, skin temperature, moisture, and neurologic status.

- Take x-rays before and after reduction is performed.

- Immobilize the shoulder with a sling and swath bandage.

Hip Dislocation

Dislocation of a hip is a serious injury and is considered an orthopedic emergency. The dislocation may be anterior or posterior and is seen in all age groups.

Mechanism of injury is usually secondary to major trauma. For example, in head-on auto crashes when the leg is extended with the foot on the break pedal or when the knee is jammed into the dashboard at the time of impact, and the resulting force dislocates the hip (see Figure 10-2). The complaint is of pain in the hip. Signs include a hip that is flexed, adducted and internally rotated with posterior dislocation, or flexed, abducted, and externally rotated with anterior dislocation. The patient cannot move his leg and his hip feels locked.

FIGURE 10-2: DISLOCATED HIP

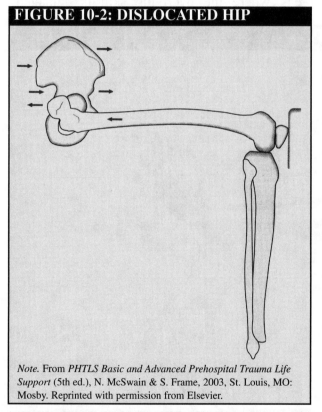

Note. From *PHTLS Basic and Advanced Prehospital Trauma Life Support* (5th ed.), N. McSwain & S. Frame, 2003, St. Louis, MO: Mosby. Reprinted with permission from Elsevier.

- The patient's hip should be manually reduced promptly upon arrival in the emergency department.

- Splint the hip in the position of greatest comfort.

- Identify all other injuries.

- Maintain bed rest after reduction.

- Treat children with a spica cast.

Posterior hip dislocation can cause sciatic nerve injury and permanent disability. Other complications are femoral artery and nerve damage. Blood supply to the femoral head may be impaired and cause avascular necrosis if the dislocation is not reduced within 6 hours. In this situation, a hip replacement will be necessary.

Knee Dislocation

Generally the result of major trauma, knee dislocations are seen in all age groups. Types are anterior, posterior, medial, lateral, or rotary.

The patient has severe knee pain, swelling, deformity, and cannot move the leg.

- Immediately splint the limb in the presenting position or the position of most comfort to the patient.

- Knee dislocations urgently need reduction and immobilization. Treatment is a splint or hinged brace.

- The patient should be on bed rest after reduction, with the leg elevated and intermittent cold packs applied for about one week.

- Arterial assessment is a high priority.

- Injury to the popliteal artery occurs in about one quarter of the cases because the artery can become caught between the adductor hiatus proximally and the interosseous membrane distally.

- Arteriography or immediate operation is necessary if there is unequal neurovascular evaluation. There is a risk of undetected arterial injury with late occlusion in knee dislocations. Therefore, even though there may not be any signs of arterial damage, arteriography should be considered.

- Tibial, popliteal, and peroneal nerve injuries are common in knee dislocations, as are fractures of the tibia.

Fractures

A broken bone is a fracture. The fracture may be open or closed (see Figure 10-3). The fracture may be direct (occurring at the point of impact) or indirect (occurring at a distance from where the force is applied). An example of indirect fracture is when a person falls on an outstretched arm and the fracture is in the clavicle. In other situations, a sudden, violent contraction of a muscle may fracture the associated bone.

CLASSIFICATIONS OF FRACTURES

Fractures (see Figure 10-4) are classified with respect to the following

- **Integrity of the skin:** Open or closed

- **Pattern:** Transverse, oblique, spiral, greenstick, impacted, compression, depressed, avulsion

- **Morphology:** Simple (two parts) and comminuted (three or more parts)

- **Location:** Proximal, middle or distal; extra-articular or intra-articular

- **Radiographic parameters:** Displacement, angulation, rotation, shortening, apposition

The most important factor in the assessment of a fracture is the integrity of the skin over the break and the surrounding soft tissues. The degree of soft tissue damage in closed or open fractures is important. Extensive soft tissue injury increases the risk of compartment syndrome.

Open or compound fracture is any bone break where the overlying skin is damaged.

FIGURE 10-3: OPEN AND CLOSED FRACTURES

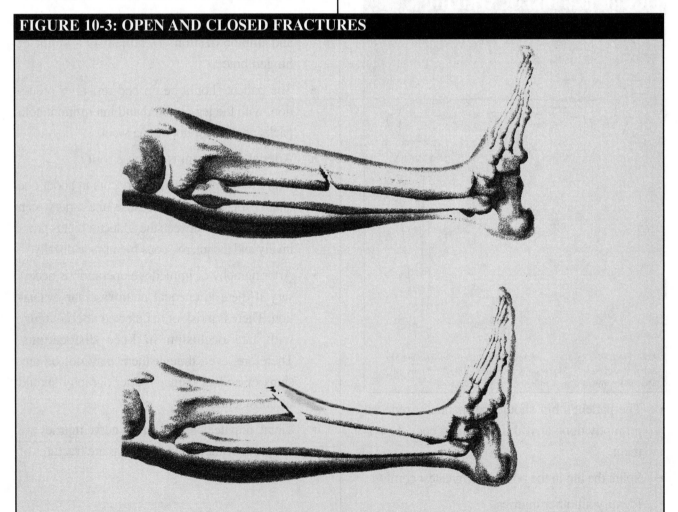

Note. From *Prehospital Emergency Care*, by J.J. Mistovich, B.Q. Hafen, and K.J. Karren, 2004, Upper Saddle River, NJ: Prentice Hall. Reprinted with permission.

FIGURE 10-4: FRACTURE PATTERN TYPES

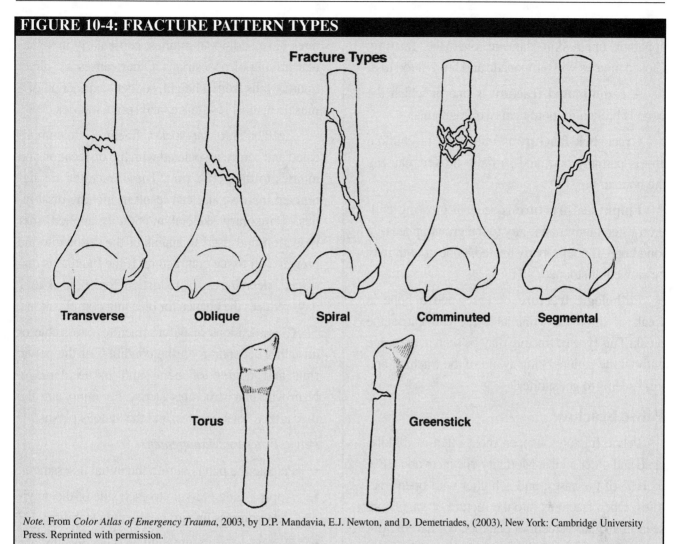

Fracture Types

Transverse   Oblique   Spiral   Comminuted   Segmental

Torus   Greenstick

Note. From *Color Atlas of Emergency Trauma*, 2003, by D.P. Mandavia, E.J. Newton, and D. Demetriades, (2003), New York: Cambridge University Press. Reprinted with permission.

Laceration may occur when the bone ends protrude through the skin or when the skin is broken from the exterior at the time of the injury. The wound may vary in size from small to gaping with exposed bone and soft tissue. The broken bone does not have to be visible in the wound to be considered an open fracture. Open fractures are more serious than closed because of the potential for hemorrhage, shock, foreign bodies, and infection (see Table 10-1). Infections can cause long-term problems for the patient. For this reason, open fractures are considered surgically urgent.

Wound care includes sterile saline irrigation, sterile dressing, IV fluid replacement, antibiotics, and analgesia. Wound cultures should be done before irrigation is begun.

TABLE 10-1: BLOOD LOSS CAUSED BY FRACTURES

Fracture	Blood Loss (ml)
Humerus	500-1,500
Elbow	250-750
Radius	250-500
Pelvis	750-6,000
Femur	500-3,000
Tibia/Fibula	250-2,000
Ankle	250-1,000

(DeDoer, Mintjes-deGroot, & Severignem, 1999)

A **closed fracture** is a bone break with no apparent open skin damage over the fracture. Closed injuries will tamponade and limit blood loss.

A **comminuted fracture** is one in which the bone is broken in more than two fragments.

Greenstick fracture is only seen in children and is partially bent and partially broken, causing the bone to bow.

Epiphyseal fracture is seen in growing children when there is an injury to the growth plate of a long bone. If not properly treated, bone growth may be slowed or stopped.

Pathologic fracture occurs when a bone is weak or diseased. Minimal force can cause the break. This type of fracture may be seen in the spine without the patient being aware of the fracture, and just "seems to get shorter."

Pelvic Fracture

Pelvic fractures happen most often in middle-aged and older adults. Mortality occurs in about 8% to 10% of the cases; and is higher with open fractures. Open fractures into the rectum or vagina are seen in a small percent of patients, but have a 50% risk of mortality (Peitzman at al., 2002). Side impact MVCs are also a common cause of severe pelvic fractures (see Figure 10-5).

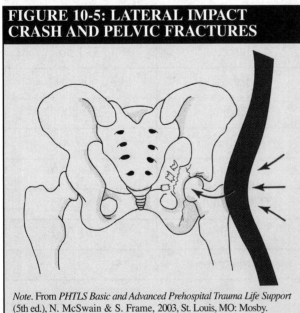

FIGURE 10-5: LATERAL IMPACT CRASH AND PELVIC FRACTURES

Note. From *PHTLS Basic and Advanced Prehospital Trauma Life Support* (5th ed.), N. McSwain & S. Frame, 2003, St. Louis, MO: Mosby. Reprinted with permission from Elsevier.

More than half of the patients with pelvic fractures have additional injuries, particularly in vehicular trauma of pedestrians. Other causes are direct trauma, falls from a height, sudden contraction of a muscle against resistance, and sports injuries.

Acetabular, or hip socket, fractures are complicated and can be associated with hip dislocation and injuries to the pelvic ring. These fractures are significant injuries, and can result in lifelong disabilities. Temporary skeletal traction is applied after reduction and used to maintain the reduction and prevent soft tissue contracture. If the fracture is displaced, delaying open reduction for about 3 to 7 days reduces the chance for bleeding complications.

Classifications of pelvic fractures are stable or unstable, depending on the condition of the pelvic ring and degree of bone and tissue damage. Neurovascular structures at risk for injury are the iliac artery, sciatic nerve, and the venous plexus.

Pelvic Fracture Management

• Palpate the pelvis during the initial assessment.

• Apply gentle pressure to each side of the pelvis and compress inward to ascertain stability.

• Compression should only be done once by one clinician and accurately documented.

• Repeated manipulation of pelvic fractures is to be avoided as they tend to bleed profusely and continued movement will cause increased blood loss.

• There may also be paraspinous muscle spasm, sacroiliac joint tenderness, paresis or hemiparesis, and pelvic ecchymosis.

• Interventions include high-flow oxygen, vital signs every 5 min with observation for signs of hypovolemia.

• Establish two large-bore IV lines for volume replacement.

• Placement of a commercially available pelvic binder or wrap a sheet around the pelvis closes the hips and tamponades bleeding.

• Type and crossmatch 6 units of blood.

- Perform radiographic studies as ordered.

- Insert Foley catheter if there is no blood at the meatus.

- Use external fixation with unstable weight-bearing fractures.

- Nonweight-bearing, less severe fractures are treated with bed rest and traction.

Other problems with pelvic fractures are varied and may be severe, including bladder trauma, genital trauma, lumbosacral trauma, rupture of internal organs, sepsis, shock, and death. Posttraumatic arthritis, chondrolysis, and heterotopic ossification are the most common complications. Long-term problems, aside from chronic pain and loss of function, are thrombophlebitis and fat embolism.

Femur Fracture

It takes substantial force to fracture the femur, a serious injury that usually occurs in conjunction with other musculoskeletal and soft tissue damage. Be sure to evaluate for other injuries, especially of the knee (see Figure 10-6).

Severe pain, inability to stand on the affected leg, swelling, crepitus, deformity, external rotation, or angulation indicate a femoral fracture. Shortening may develop due to severe muscle spasms.

Femur Fracture Management

- Immobilize the leg with use of a commercial traction splint.

- Check pulse and movement of toes before and after splint application.

- If pulse diminished after traction application, reduce traction and recheck pulse.

- At least one IV site should be established, with frequent vital signs and circulation checks conducted.

- Monitor hemodynamic stability. It is not unusual for approximately 2 L to bleed into the thigh.

- Immobilization with traction splint and administration of analgesia will decrease severe muscle spasms, which can move bone ends, causing

FIGURE 10-6: DASHBOARD POINTS OF IMPACT IN MVC: KNEE AND FEMUR FRACTURES

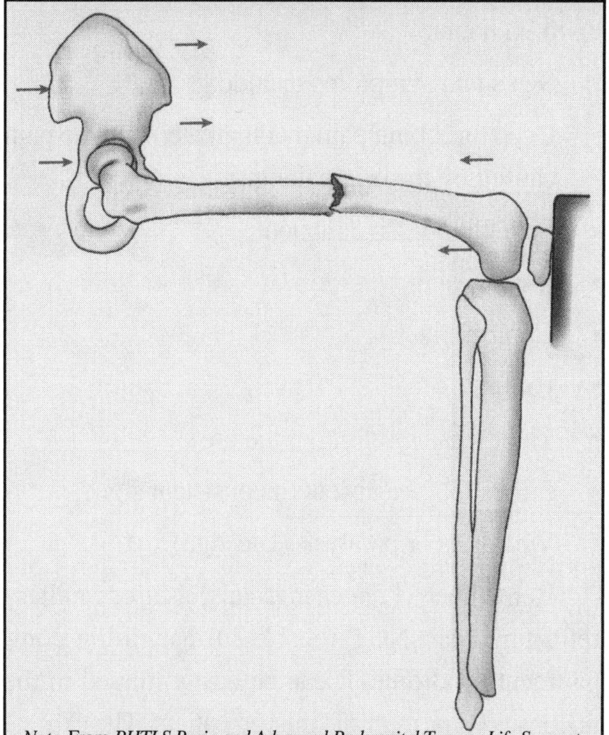

Note. From *PHTLS Basic and Advanced Prehospital Trauma Life Support* (5th ed.), N. McSwain & S. Frame, 2003, St. Louis, MO: Mosby. Reprinted with permission from Elsevier.

further soft-tissue injury, muscle damage, and pain.

- Neurovascular damage can include the peroneal and sciatic nerves and popliteal artery.

COMPLICATIONS OF FRACTURES

Fractures have several potential complications. Maintain a high index of suspicion for compartment syndrome and fat emboli when caring for patient with fractures.

Compartment Syndrome

Soft-tissue injuries, fractures, or casts can compress soft tissue causing compartment syndrome. When swelling and/or compression cause pressure in the muscle compartment to rise to the point that microvascular circulation is compromised, it is known as compartment syndrome. The result is tissue ischemia, which threatens the limb.

This syndrome is most often seen in compartments of the lower leg and forearm, with symptoms developing within 6 to 8 hours but possibly delayed up to 96 hours.

Signs and symptoms include:

- Deep throbbing pain much greater than the pain caused by the original injury
- Pain with passive flexion
- Paresthesia
- Coolness
- Pallor
- Tight tense swelling of the area
- Pulses may be absent (inconsistent sign)
- Weakness or paralysis (late sign)

Remember, changes in distal pulses or capillary refill times are NOT reliable in diagnosing compartment syndrome. It can be easily missed in the unconscious or multiple injured patient. The clinical diagnosis is based on history of injury and physical signs coupled with a high index of suspicion. The physician may perform intracompartmental pressure measurements periodically to assess tissue pressures. Pressures greater than 35 to 45 mm Hg suggest need for fasciotomy. Within 4 to 6 hours, irreversible tissue damage will occur from the inadequate perfusion. This is an urgent situation and should be identified and reported to the physician as soon as possible.

Compartment Syndrome Management

- Position the limb on the same level as the heart.
- Perform frequent neurovascular checks.
- Report all changes immediately to the physician.
- Assist the physician to perform compartment pressure checks if signs and symptoms persist.
- Prepare the patient for emergency surgery for a fasciotomy.

Fat Embolism

Fat embolism is an unusual but life-threatening complication. It becomes apparent 24 to 48 hours after bone injury. This complication is seen most often with pelvic, femoral, or tibia fractures. When a fracture occurs, it causes the release of fat particles into the blood. These particles may embolize to the lungs, signaled by sudden tachycardia, tachypnea, shortness of breath, cyanosis, cough, temperature elevation, altered level of consciousness, and pulmonary edema leading to acute respiratory distress syndrome.

Traumatic Amputations

Amputation trauma has the potential of significant morbidity. Dysfunctional limbs should be treated at facilities with the capability of microvascular surgery. This trauma is threatening to the patient's life and limbs, is a true emergency, and treatment must be immediate. Partial amputations tend to bleed more than complete amputations.

Mechanisms of injury are most frequently industrial or recreational accidents. Lawn mowers and snowblowers also cause a large number of amputations.

The most frequently amputated body parts are fingers and toes, distal half of the foot, leg, forearm, hand, ear, nose, and penis.

Traumatic Amputation Management

- High-flow oxygen, two large-bore IV lines and control of bleeding are top priorities.
- Splint and support the limb in a position of anatomic function if the amputation is partial.
- In total amputations, the stump should be elevated, irrigated with sterile saline, and sterile dressings applied.
- Orders will include antibiotics, tetanus booster, and immune globulin.
- Tourniquets should not be applied unless ordered by the physician.

- The amputated part should be brought with the patient to the emergency department for possible reimplantation.

- The amputated part should be wrapped in sterile gauze, wet with saline, and placed in a watertight plastic bag or container, which is then put in a container with iced saline.

- Do not use dry ice or distilled water, or place the amputated part directly on ice or allow it to freeze, as it will damage the tissue.

- Label the container with the patient's name, time, and date.

Success of reimplantation is extremely limited. The availability of a reimplantation team, the type and degree of damage to the stump and amputated part, and the amount of time that has passed since the incident are the key factors in the success of reimplantation. Other factors are age, general physical condition, occupation, and motivation.

Amputations caused by sharp cuts have a better outcome than crush injuries and avulsions.

Occult Injuries

Occult injuries are those injuries that are hidden, under appreciated, or are missed on initial assessment. They are frequently minor musculoskeletal injuries that were overlooked when initially dealing with the more life-threatening injuries. Many patients do not initially complain of these more minor injuries when dealing with the distracting pain of major injuries, or they may be unconscious making identification even more difficult. Therefore it is imperative to repeatedly reevaluate the patient to assess for these musculoskeletal injuries. Some of these injuries may not be identified until up to days after admission.

Prioritizing Orthopedic Emergencies

Most orthopedic injuries are not emergencies. Other life-threatening emergencies always take precedence. However there are orthopedic injuries that require immediate management:

1. **Hip dislocations** (due to potential impaired blood supply and resulting in avascular necrosis with permanent disability – a true orthopedic emergency)

   — Physician to reduce promptly

2. **Knee dislocations** (due to potential vascular disruption)

   — Prompt arteriogram required and surgery if necessary

3. **Open fractures** (due to infection and osteomyelitis)

   — To operating room for wash out by an orthopedic surgeon within 6 hours of injury

4. **Massive pelvic fractures** (due to hemodynamic instability)

   — Apply pelvic binder to tamponade blood loss

   — Prompt evaluation/transfer to an orthopedic surgeon

ASSESSMENT PRINCIPLES

As discussed in the previous chapters, the ABC assessment and maintenance is always the first priority. It is important not to allow dramatic orthopedic injuries to distract from more serious trauma.

Rapid assessment follows the ABCs to identify serious injuries of the head, cervical spine, chest, and abdomen and identify the prioritization of actions. Musculoskeletal injuries are not isolated in serious traumatic incidents.

- Intervene in life-threatening injuries first, limb-threatening injuries second, and then other injuries according to severity. Injured nerves and vessels have the potential for causing permanent disability.

- Obtain as accurate a history as possible while examining the patient. Ascertain any previous musculoskeletal injuries, diseases, or surgeries.

- Do not pull off the patient's clothing, but cut it away, being careful not to disturb the injured area and always protecting the patient's privacy.

- Assess for open wounds and skin integrity, checking for internal as well as external bleeding.

- Compare the injured extremity with the opposite limb, checking for pain, point tenderness, swelling, discoloration, and temperature.

- Palpate injured areas gently, feeling for irregularities and signs of dislocations and fractures.

- If the patient is a child, look for indicators of abuse when the patient has a spiral fracture.

- Palpate for pulses distally and in both extremities; compare extremities.

- Assess neurovascular status, checking for numbness and paresthesia. Determine if the patient can wiggle his fingers or toes.

- Assess the circulatory status of extremities.

MANAGEMENT PRINCIPLES

Remember that with major trauma, there will be multiple injuries. The primary goal is to limit current damage, prevent further damage, and preserve the structure and function of the injured extremity as much as possible.

- Conduct the ABCs and immobilize the neck until cervical injury has been cleared.

- If the patient has multiple severe injuries, a long bone fracture or possible pelvic fracture, provide 100% oxygen and administer IV fluids to keep the patient adequately perfused, as hypovolemic shock is likely.

- Provide adequate sedation and analgesia prior to manual reduction of fractures. Carefully monitor the airway and vital signs during conscious sedation. Continuously monitor the pulse oximetry and keep necessary emergency airway equipment at the bedside.

- If there is an open wound, culture if ordered, gently irrigate with sterile saline solution and cover with a sterile dressing. Do not spread the wound apart to determine its depth.

- Do not apply a tourniquet unless ordered by the physician.

- Give nothing-by-mouth until the physician determines that surgical intervention is not necessary or if the patient is nauseated.

- Maintain patient temperature to avoid hypothermia.

- Reassess the injured limb serially and after each time the limb has been moved.

- Splint the injured extremity above and below the injury site.

- Check pulse before and after splint application.

- If pulse is lost after traction is applied, release the traction and reassess pulse.

- Do not attempt to straighten a dislocated or fractured limb. If not already splinted, immobilize the limb in the most comfortable position or as the limb presents.

- Immobilizing fractures assists in pain control by reducing movement.

- Do not attempt to remove any impaled object; stabilize the object until the physician arrives for trauma management.

- Exposed bones should not be pushed back into the wound; it will aggravate the injury, increase the potential for infection, and be painful.

- If there is an amputation, transport the amputated part to the emergency department with the patient. It is not advisable to suggest to the patient that reimplantation is usually successful. It is not.

- If the amputation is partial, the limb should be supported and splinted in a position of anatomic function. Assess hemodynamic stability frequently as partial amputations bleed more aggressively than complete amputations.

- A full amputation should have the stump gently irrigated for gross contamination, a sterile dressing applied, and it should be elevated.

- The amputated part should be wrapped in sterile gauze, wet with saline solution. Place in a water-tight plastic bag or container, which should then be put in a container with iced saline solution.

- Do not use dry ice or distilled water or place the amputated part directly on ice or allow to freeze as it will damage the tissue. Label the container with the patient's name, time, and date.

- Amputated parts should not be soaked in any liquid, cleaned, or rinsed. Doing so would ruin the integrity of the tissue.

- Prevent acute renal failure in rhabdomyolysis with aggressive fluid resuscitation (initially to maintain urine output at 100 ml/hour), osmotic diuretics, and alkalization of the urine.

CASE STUDY

A 43-year-old female sustained a head-on motorcycle crash collision with a tree. At the scene, she was combative, systolic blood pressure was 80 mm Hg, heart rate 122 beats/min and respiratory rate 24 breaths/min. In the emergency department, her vital signs have improved to normal and the patient is complaining of pain in her right arm and both legs. There is marked deformity of the right thigh and left lower extremity. Emergency Medical Services (EMS) report a large laceration to the left leg which now has a dressing over it.

Answer the following case study questions, writing your responses on a separate sheet of paper. Compare your responses to the answers that follow:

1. List the initial nursing assessment priorities.

2. Identify the initial assessment of an extremity for injury.

3. Explain how to assess for occult orthopedic injury.

4. Define the steps for immobilization of extremity injuries.

5. Define the steps for reevaluation of extremity injuries.

Answers

1. Check vital signs and ABCs first (primary survey). Confirm that the patient is hemodynamically normal before beginning the secondary survey, which is where musculoskeletal assessment occurs.

2. Examine the patient's injured extremities. Assess neurovascular status of each extremity by checking the distal pulse, movement, and sensation.

3. Assess for any open wounds, clean them, and apply a dressing.

4. Immobilize each injured extremity by splinting. Immobilization prevents further soft tissue injury, and contributes to hemorrhage control and pain relief.

5. Reevaluate neurovascular status (pulse check and movement) after manipulation and application of splints.

SUMMARY

A large portion of the trauma patients seen in emergency departments have musculoskeletal injuries. Most of these injuries are not threatening to the patient's life or limbs, although orthopedic trauma with associated neurovascular damage is a significant cause of short- and long-term disabilities. Orthopedic trauma includes soft-tissue injuries, dislocations, fractures, and traumatic amputations. There may be multiple injuries in addition to the musculoskeletal trauma.

The primary objective for emergency care of orthopedic trauma is to restore or preserve the injured limb with the greatest integrity possible and prevent further injury. Quick and appropriate evaluation and intervention may prevent disability.

EXAM QUESTIONS

CHAPTER 10

Questions 61-66

61. What do tendons connect?

    a. Muscle to bone

    b. Bone to bone

    c. Muscle to muscle

    d. Cartilage to cartilage

62. A 56-year-old farmer is found trapped from the waist down beneath his overturned tractor. He has been pinned for 4 hours prior to being found. He is hemodynamically unstable. He is awake and alert until just before arriving to the emergency department. He is now losing consciousness and responds only to painful stimuli by moaning. His pupils are 3 mm in diameter, symmetrical, and reactive to light. EMS report that he could not move his legs even with painful stimuli. The most likely cause of his deterioration is

    a. intracerebral hemorrhage.

    b. central cord syndrome.

    c. pelvic fracture associated hemorrhage.

    d. bilateral leg compartment syndrome.

63. Which of the following dislocations is considered a true orthopedic emergency?

    a. Hip dislocation

    b. Compound fracture of the leg

    c. Shoulder dislocation

    d. Elbow dislocation

64. Which of the following statements regarding assessment of compartment syndrome are true?

    a. The distal pulse will be absent.

    b. It commonly occurs in the upper thigh and lower leg muscles.

    c. It can be easily identified in the head injured patient.

    d. The patient's complaint of pain is out of proportion to the injury.

65. Initial nursing assessment management of musculoskeletal injuries includes

    a. splint the extremity first prior to assessing for injury.

    b. assess integrity of the skin over the point of injury and surrounding tissues to determine if a closed or open fracture.

    c. pull off the patient's clothing as fast as possible if a fracture with hemorrhage is suspected.

    d. straighten the limb prior to splint application.

66. A 50-year-old man sustains a closed femur fracture in an MVC. The left thigh is angulated. A traction splint is applied to the injured leg and shortly afterward the patient complains of severe pain in his foot and lower leg. Assessment reveals absent pedal pulses. The appropriate nursing intervention is to

    a. elevate the extremity.

    b. administer pain medication.

    c. release traction.

    d. tighten the traction.

CHAPTER 11

BURN AND COLD TRAUMA

CHAPTER OBJECTIVE

Upon completion of this chapter, the reader will be able to describe the concepts important in the management of burn and cold injuries.

LEARNING OBJECTIVES

Upon completion of this chapter, the reader should be able to

1. identify the normal functions of the skin.

2. identify the pathophysiology of burn injuries.

3. identify types of burn and cold injuries and the criteria for describing the extent and severity of those injuries.

4. identify appropriate basic nursing interventions for the burn patient.

5. identify appropriate basic interventions for the cold injury patient.

INTRODUCTION

Burn and cold injuries comprise major causes of morbidity and mortality. Attention to basic principles of trauma care and timely application of emergency measures should minimize complications from these injuries. Principles such as high index of suspicion for airway compromise, smoke inhalation, and potential hemodynamic instability will in large part prevent unnecessary morbidity and mortality. An awareness of potential complications such as rhabdomyolysis, hypothermia, and cardiac dysrhythmias is necessary to avoid morbidity.

The majority of burns are preventable. Because of recent strong public education programs and legislative mandate regarding construction codes and smoke/fire detection devices, efforts are met with increasing effectiveness in decreasing the number of burn injuries.

EPIDEMIOLOGY

Residential fires are the main cause of burn deaths, with the predominant mechanisms being heating unit failure, kitchen accidents, incendiary devices/arson, and smoking materials.

In the home, scalding most often causes pediatric burns. They may be unintentional or deliberate, and it takes careful observation and history taking to determine if the child's burn is the result of abuse.

High-risk groups for fire incidents include those who smoke, especially in bed; children; older adults; and disabled people.

Fire is not the only source of burns. Electricity, including lightening; ultraviolet rays; superheated steam; chemicals; tar; explosions; and frostbite are also mechanisms that cause burns.

ANATOMY AND FUNCTIONS OF SKIN

Skin is the largest single organ in the body, and as a true organ, it has functions. Three major functions are to **protect** the body in the environment, **regulate** the temperature of the body, and **transmit** information about the environment to the brain. In other words, the skin protects, regulates, and informs.

LAYERS OF THE SKIN

Epidermis

Of the two main layers of skin, the epidermis is the tough outermost layer (see Figure 11-1). There are several layers within the epidermis. The base epidermal layer is the germinal layer, which continuously produces new cells that rise to the surface, die, and form the watertight covering. The epidermis varies in thickness in different parts of the body.

Dermis

A deeper layer, the dermis, is below the germinal layer and consists of collagen and elastic fibers. Within the dermis are specialized structures that give the skin its characteristic appearance: sweat glands, sebaceous glands that secrete oil to lubricate the skin, hair follicles, blood vessels, and specialized nerve endings.

Subcutaneous Tissue

Lying below the dermis, subcutaneous tissue is the fatty layer that varies in thickness in different parts of the body and in each person.

Fascia

Below the subcutaneous layer lies the deepest layer, the fascia, which covers the muscles.

FIGURE 11-1: THREE-DIMENSIONAL SECTION OF THE SKIN

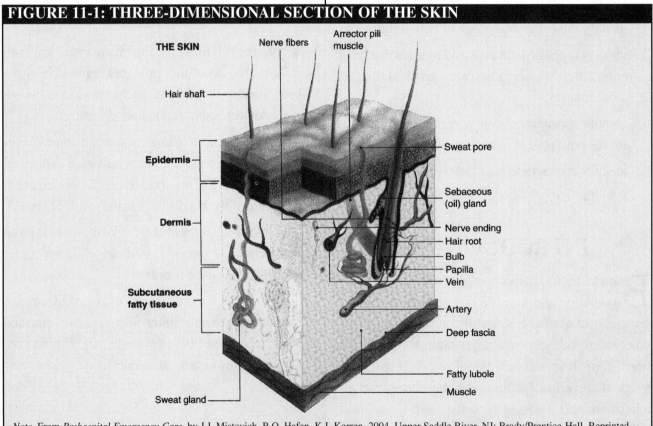

Note. From *Prehospital Emergency Care*, by J.J. Mistovich, B.Q. Hafen, K.J. Karren, 2004, Upper Saddle River, NJ: Brady/Prentice-Hall. Reprinted with permission.

FUNCTIONS

Protection

The skin is watertight. More than 70% of the body is made up of water containing an exact balance of chemical substances in its solution. The watertight quality of the skin keeps the balance of the internal water solution stable. The body is also protected from the invasion of infectious organisms, bacteria, viruses, and fungi, as they cannot pass through unbroken skin.

Regulation

Skin is the major organ in the body for temperature regulation. The metabolic processes can only function within a narrow temperature range. If the temperature is too low, reactions cannot occur, metabolism stops, and the body dies. If the temperature is too high, the rate of metabolism increases, sometimes resulting in permanent tissue damage and death.

When the environment is cold, constriction of the blood vessels shunts the blood away from the skin's surface to decrease the amount of heat radiated. When the environment is hot, sweat is secreted to the skin's surface for evaporation. Evaporation of sweat uses energy, which is taken from the body as heat, causing the body temperature to fall. In other words, sweating itself does not reduce the body temperature; it is the process of evaporation pulling energy from the body in the form of heat that reduces the temperature.

Information

Sensory nerves originating in the skin carry information about the environment to the brain, including sensations of pressure, pleasant stimuli, and pain.

PATHOPHYSIOLOGY

The generally accepted definition of a burn is that it occurs when the skin is exposed to more energy than it can absorb. There are many causes of burns, but local and systemic responses are similar in all cases.

Zones of Damage

When a burn occurs, it causes three concentric circles or zones of damage similar in shape to a shooting target (Moore et al., 2004) (see Figure 11-2).

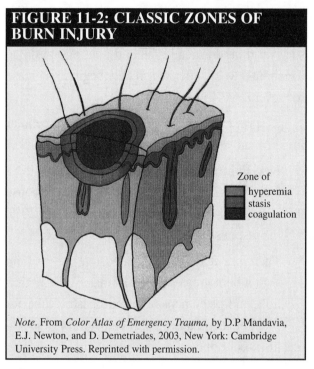

FIGURE 11-2: CLASSIC ZONES OF BURN INJURY

Zone of
hyperemia
stasis
coagulation

Note. From *Color Atlas of Emergency Trauma*, by D.P Mandavia, E.J. Newton, and D. Demetriades, 2003, New York: Cambridge University Press. Reprinted with permission.

Zone 1

The zone of coagulation: This is the inner most circle or central zone of coagulation. This is the burn area of deepest injury with often-irreversible damage.

Zone 2

The zone of stasis: This is the next outer ring of injured area where capillary and small vessel stasis (stagnation of the normal flow of fluids, in this case, blood) occurs and surrounds zone 1. The outcome of the burn wound depends upon resolution or progression of this area of stasis. Edema formation and continued compromise of blood flow to this zone will cause a deeper and more extensive wound. When there is decreased perfusion to the skin, it can convert the zone of stasis to one of coagulation, causing the burn to become deeper. Because of this, final determination of the depth and severity of burn wound may not be known for 3 to 5 days.

Zone 3

The zone of hyperemia: This is the outermost zone or area of superficial damage that heals quickly. After a burn, there is immediate hemolysis of red blood cells; the remaining red cells have their life span reduced by about one third. Platelet count and survival time drastically fall and continue to do so for about a week, after which they begin to increase for several weeks.

Response to a burn is tissue damage, cellular impairment, and fluid shifts.

- **Key Point:** In a burn involving less than 20% total body surface area (TBSA), burn response is usually limited to the burn area. Beyond 20%, the response goes from local to systemic.

- Therefore it is recommended that any patient with a burn greater than 20% receive IV hydration, and placement of an nasogastric tube for probable ileus, and a Foley catheter for fluid status monitoring.

VASCULAR RESPONSE

After a burn occurs, there is a brief decrease in blood flow to the burned area. Then there is a marked increase in arteriole vasodilation. The burned tissues release mediators that cause an inflammatory response. Release of the vasoactive substances along with the vasodilation increase capillary permeability, or the ability of the capillary wall to let substances in the blood move back and forth into tissue spaces or cells. As a result, there is intravascular fluid loss and wound edema.

Increased capillary permeability also causes hypoproteinemia that aggravates edema in tissue that is not burned. Insensible fluid loss increases the basal metabolic rate that coupled with the fluid shift causes hypovolemia.

The capillary permeability increase maximizes in the first 24 to 48 hours and returns to normal at approximately 36 hours when there is a massive diuresis.

During the increased capillary permeability, vascular fluid shifts into the interstitium (between cells or tissues) making the blood more viscous. The decreased intravascular fluid volume, increased blood viscosity, and increase in peripheral resistance contribute to a decrease in cardiac output. The drop in cardiac output and blood volume and the sympathetic nervous system response of shunting blood to the heart and brain decreases perfusion to the skin, viscera, and kidneys. The drop in circulating plasma along with the increased hematocrit may lead to hemoglobinuria and renal failure if the patient is not appropriately fluid resuscitated.

Serious burn injury may affect all the body organs. Cerebral perfusion abnormalities, impaired cardiac blood supply, renal insufficiency, and metabolic imbalance are likely consequences of large and or deep burns.

PULMONARY RESPONSE TO SMOKE INHALATION

Smoke inhalation results in three possible injuries (American College of Surgeons, 2004a):

1. Carbon monoxide intoxication

2. Upper airway obstruction

3. Chemical damage to the lower airways and lung parenchyma

Carbon Monoxide Intoxication

The most frequent cause of death in fire occurs in victims who have been overcome by carbon monoxide before they are burned. Carbon monoxide is a colorless, odorless gas released during a fire, and when inhaled and absorbed, it binds with hemoglobin, displacing oxygen and blocking oxygen-binding sites. Carbon monoxide has an affinity for hemoglobin that is 200 times greater than that of oxygen. When carbon monoxide binds to hemoglobin, it interferes with adequate amounts of oxygen getting to the tissues. Additionally, carbon monoxide combines with myoglobin in the muscle cells, causing muscle weakness. The tissue hypoxia that results in muscle weakness and mental confusion is thought to be a primary contributor to fatalities. The signs and symptoms of poisoning depend on the level of carbon monoxide, the length of exposure, and the individual's health condition.

- Early in carbon monoxide poisoning, while in the fire situation or just after, the patient feels few symptoms that he or she perceives as serious: some muscle weakness and mild dyspnea. The patient may become confused.

- Later signs of carbon monoxide poisoning are pink to cherry red skin, tachycardia, tachypnea, headache, dizziness, and nausea.

- Blood gases should be drawn to measure the level of carboxyhemoglobin, the compound formed by carbon monoxide and hemoglobin in carbon monoxide poisoning.

- Levels of carboxyhemoglobin below 15% rarely have symptoms and are often seen in heavy smokers. Symptoms such as headache and confusion are seen in levels ranging from 15-40%.

- Greater than 40% blood levels may result in coma. If the patient is thought to have carbon monoxide poisoning, 100% oxygen should be given.

Upper Airway Obstruction

Thermal injury to the upper airway is usually related to facial burns. Intrinsic or extrinsic edema may occlude the airway at the level of the vocal cords or higher. Edema progresses rapidly, causing total occlusion within minutes to hours.

Tissue damage in the posterior pharynx is usually from thermal causes. It is not likely that thermal damage occurs below the posterior pharynx because this area is an efficient system for heat exchange. When there is true thermal injury below the vocal cords, it is usually caused by superheated steam carried by water vapor into the lungs, or the inhalation of explosive gases. Immediate early intubation is required. If there is any doubt prophylactic intubation is preferred.

Chemical Injury

Smoke inhalation often causes chemical injury to the lower airways and lung parenchyma. Carbon particles contained in smoke travel down to the bronchi and into the alveoli.

Chemical injury causes hemorrhagic tracheobronchitis, an increase in edema, lowered levels of surfactant, and decreased function of pulmonary cells that are dust-phagocytic (macrophages). Generally within 24 to 48 hours, acute respiratory distress syndrome (ARDS) begins to develop.

In the case of severe inhalation injury, the patient will have an increased need for fluids.

MECHANISM OF INJURY

Burns, the application of more energy than the body can absorb without damage, occur in several forms:

1. Thermal heat – flame, scalds, contact, steam, and flash

2. Chemical – including contact and inhalation

3. Electrical – including shock and lightning

4. Nuclear radiation – ionizing radiation and nuclear radiation

Damage to the body ranges from minor to fatal. Accidents, motor vehicle crashes (MVCs), and industrial and residential accidents are the greatest sources of burns. For the most part, the longer the patient is in contact with the burning agent, the more severe the burn. The type and temperature of the agent inflicting the burn also affects the degree and extent of the resulting damage. If the patient has received other additional injuries, they may complicate the patient's recovery or contribute to his death.

Thermal Burns

The majority of all burn injury, thermal or heat, mechanisms are flame, scalds, contact, steam, and flash burns. The seriousness of the burn is determined by five factors: Evaluating the depth/damage to the skin; calculating the TBSA; involvement of critical areas (hands, feet, face, genitalia); patient's age (very young or very old), the patient's general health, and additional trauma status.

Burn depth is commonly referred to by the lay public as first-, second-, and third-degree burn. Burn professionals reference the burn thickness as superficial, partial, and full-thickness. As stated before, burn depth assessment at admission is only an estimate, and the actual identification of the burn severity may take 3 to 5 days because of the evolving status of zone 2, stasis.

Scald Burns

Scalds are the most common of all burns. Water at 140° F (60° C) for 3 seconds will cause a deep partial or full-thickness burn. Liquid temperature of 156° F (69° C) will cause the same burn in only 1 seconds. To illustrate with everyday liquids used in the home, just-brewed coffee is 180° F (82° C), as are soups and sauces. Liquids of thick consistency stick to the skin longer and, therefore, burn longer. Cooking oil and grease can reach temperatures of up to 400° F (204° C).

In the case of an immersion burn, such as a bath, even though the water may be cooler than 140° F (60° C), the contact with the skin lasts longer.

Flame Burns

The second most frequent cause of burns is flames. While residential fires have decreased due to public education, detectors, and improved fire codes, still careless smoking, clothing ignited by stoves or space heaters, and MVCs still contribute to a significant number of flame burns. Outdoor

flame burns are often secondary to improper use of camping stoves, smoking in a sleeping bag, use of lanterns in tents, and the use of gasoline or kerosene on a charcoal fire.

Flash Burns

Explosions of natural gas, propane, gasoline, or other flammable liquids cause flash burns. There is brief, intense heat. The burns are mostly partial-thickness, but the depth of the burn is related to the amount and kind of fuel involved.

Contact Burns

Direct contact with a hot object can cause a deep burn. Examples of mechanisms of injury are machine-press burns, often also associated with crush injuries; hot tar; hot tools; and burners on a stove. Children may put their hand on a stove burner, hot steam iron, curling iron, or hair dryer.

Chemical Burns

Chemicals cause denaturing of the protein (protein loses some of its chemical and physical properties, just as cooking an egg white denatures the albumen) in tissues, or a desiccation (drying) of the cells. In chemical burns, the type of chemical, concentration, and length of time of exposure all affect the extent of the burn.

Acid versus Alkali Burn

Strong acids or alkalis coming in direct contact with the skin or through clothing cause most chemical burns. Alkali burns cause more damage than acids because they are corrosive and are able to combine with water. With their ability to combine with water and action on fatty acids, alkaline burns cause rapid, deep destruction of tissue. Tissue is "gelatinized," turning grayish in color, with a soapy, slippery feel.

While acids can be washed off the skin's surface, alkalis combine with the water and continue burning until the chemical itself is totally removed from the patient. If the alkali is powdered, such as lime, it should be brushed off the skin before beginning to flush. A dry alkali chemical activated by the addition of water will cause more damage to the skin than when dry.

In order to stop the chemical burning process, the chemical has to be removed from the areas of contact with the patient.

Treatment of Chemical Burns

• Brush off all powders or particles prior to flushing.

• Flooding of the area should begin as soon as possible unless there is a specific antidote available per Material Safety Data (MSD) information.

• Contain all water used for flushing, do not allow to empty into the general drainage system.

• Patient's clothing should be removed immediately, taking care not to get the chemical on the caregiver.

• Flushing should continue for at least 10 min to ensure the entire chemical is removed.

• Periodically assess the pH with a litmus test until neutral.

• Following the flushing, cover the burned area with sterile, dry dressings.

Electrical Burns

Electric Shock

Electrical burns are caused by low- or high-voltage contact, ranging from ordinary household current to utility power lines. Most electrical burns in the home are from the careless use of appliances or faulty equipment. Small children stick their fingers into electrical outlets or bite into electrical cords. Storms downing power lines that are lying in water or across an automobile is another example of electrical contact.

In order to cause a burn, electricity must enter the body at one point and exit at another point. As electricity passes through the body, it meets resistance from the body tissues and is converted to heat.

The heat generated is in direct proportion to the amperage of the current and the electrical resistance of the body parts.

As electricity passes through the skin, it leaves a burn at the entry and exit sites. There may be extensive internal injury between these sites. The amount of internal tissue injury is usually more extensive than indicated by the appearance of the skin wound. Severe damage may be done to the deeper tissues.

The heart, lungs, and brain can be damaged immediately after the body receives a shock. A burn may be followed by cardiac arrest due to a disruption in the normal electrical rhythm of the heart. Nerves, blood vessels, and muscles are less resistant and more likely to be damaged than bone or fat. The nervous system is particularly vulnerable to electrical burns. Damage to the brain, spinal cord, and myelin-producing cells can cause transverse myelitis, an acute form of myelitis involving the entire thickness of the spinal cord.

Electric current may cause violent muscle contractions resulting in fractures or dislocations. The shock may also cause the patient to fall to the ground and incur additional injury. High-voltage electricity can cause such severe destruction to muscles and skin that amputation is necessary.

Cardiopulmonary resuscitation (CPR) may be the first intervention necessary with a patient who has sustained an electrical shock. If CPR is not necessary, further interventions can be initiated. Dry, sterile dressings should be placed on the burn wounds, and fractures should be immobilized. Further burn and trauma management is relative to the damage the patient has incurred.

Lightning

Lightning is a specific form of electrical burn. It has a force of thousands of volts. The strike lasts only for a fraction of a second and is not always fatal. The high-voltage lightning strike involves the whole body. A superficial characteristic burn is usually on the skin at the site of the strike, but the burn itself, is rarely deep. However, many body systems are affected, especially the nervous and cardiovascular systems.

Most persons struck by lightning are immediately knocked unconscious and have no memory of being hit. Patients may experience numbness, tingling, partial or complete paralysis, blindness, loss of hearing, difficulty speaking, or being unable to speak at all. These problems usually resolve themselves.

The greatest concern with a lightning strike is the electrical disturbance causing a severely disrupted heart rhythm leading to ventricular fibrillation or full cardiac arrest. The absence of a heartbeat indicates vigorous resuscitation attempts should begin, because an arrest caused by dysrhythmias is often reversible. Patients can be successfully resuscitated with immediate CPR and defibrillation.

Nuclear Radiation Burns

Nuclear reaction energy causes several types of injuries. Solar radiation causes burns similar to thermal burns. The heat from atomic explosions also produces burns similar to thermal burns. Exposure to radioactive chemicals and materials that result in acute burns have accompanying problems, including chronic illness or death.

Radiation Burns

Ionizing radiation from the sun passes through the ozone layer of the atmosphere and is able to cause a burn injury. The burns are not often serious and rarely worse than a first-degree burn. If a large portion of the body is affected, discomfort may develop, along with mild hypotension.

Nuclear Radiation Exposure

We are all exposed to some nuclear radiation through cosmic rays and natural radioactive materials.

Since the development of nuclear power, many people work with highly radioactive materials. Transportation of radioactive materials also provides an opportunity for accidental exposure.

The main concern regarding radiation accidents is to remove the radiation source from the patient or move the patient or patients away from the radiation source. If radioactive material has been spilled on clothing, it should be removed and stored in special containers. Then the patient should shower in a designated area. Care should be taken to contain the radioactive material.

Any other injuries should be assessed and appropriate interventions taken.

Hospitals are required to have policies and procedures regarding hazardous material treatment and disposal.

ASSESSMENT HISTORY

Concomitant Injuries

The history of the injury is important in managing the burn patient. A high index of suspicion is necessary to find associated injuries sustained while the victim attempts to escape the fire. Explosions can throw the patient resulting in internal injuries and/or fractures. It is important that the time of burn injury be established. Burns sustained within an enclosed space should suggest the potential for inhalation injury.

Preexisting Disease

History should include assessment of any preexisting disease such as cardiac, pulmonary, diabetes, hypertension, renal disease, and any medications the patient is taking. Tetanus immunization is essential to establish.

Extent

TBSA Burned

Rule of Nines: The extent or amount of body surface area affected by thermal or chemical burns is calculated by using the Rule of Nines (see Figure 11-3). Using this formula permits rapid, accurate assessment. The system divides the body into sections, each representing approximately 9% of the TBSA. Obviously, because of different body proportions, the rule is modified in infants and small children, pregnant women, and some other patients.

Electrical injuries are more difficult to evaluate, due to the fact that surface area may be considerably less than the underlying damage.

The general formula for determining the TBSA in adults:

- Each upper extremity is counted as 9%.
- Each lower extremity is considered 18%.
- The front trunk is 18%.
- The back trunk is 18%.
- Genitals and perineum are 1%.
- The palmar surface (including fingers) of the patients hand can be used to approximate 1% of the patients body surface when assessing small scattered burns.

Depth

Assess for the depth of burn, which is important in evaluating the severity of the burn, planning for wound care, and predicting functional and cosmetic results (see Figure 11-4).

First-Degree: Only the superficial epidermis is injured with minimal damage. The skin has mild erythema, no blistering, and there is no burning through the layers of skin. The epidermis may peel in small scales without scarring. Discomfort resolves in a day or two. Sunburn is a good example of a first-degree burn. This burn generally does not require IV fluid replacement.

Second-Degree: Also known as a partial-thickness burn, the entire epidermis and layers of the dermis are damaged. The entire dermis is not destroyed, nor is there damage to the subcutaneous layer. The skin is erythematous, edematous, and painful. Blisters will form. The burn heals in 7 to 14 days as the epithelial layer regenerates. Scalds most commonly are second-degree burns.

Middle and deep burns extend to the deeper dermal layers, leaving little tissue intact. They are less painful than more superficial burns because of some nerve damage, and blisters are not usually seen. The skin is reddened and has extensive weeping of plasma.

FIGURE 11-3: RULE OF NINES

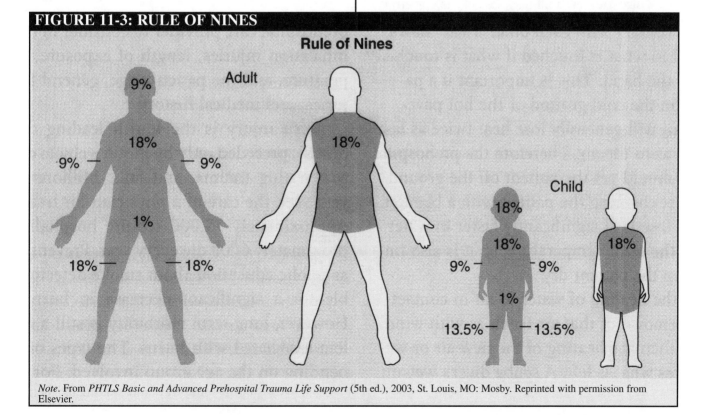

Note. From PHTLS Basic and Advanced Prehospital Trauma Life Support (5th ed.), 2003, St. Louis, MO: Mosby. Reprinted with permission from Elsevier.

FIGURE 11-4: BURN DEPTH

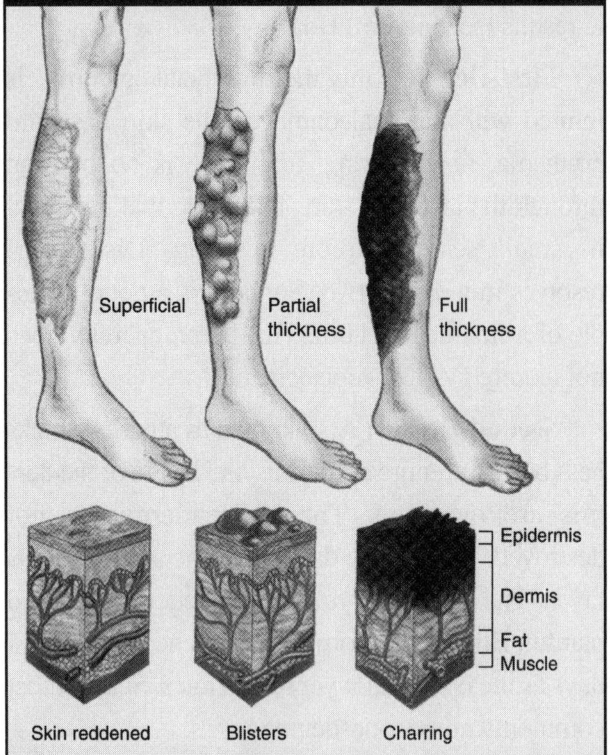

Note. From *Essentials of Emergency Care* (3rd ed.), by D. Limmer, B. Elling, and M. O'Keefe, 2002, Upper Saddle River, NJ: Prentice Hall. Reprinted with permission.

Spontaneous healing may take weeks to months to resolve, often leaving dense scarring.

Third-Degree: Full-thickness of the epidermis and dermis is destroyed, and damage may extend through or beyond the subcutaneous fat. The burned area may appear waxy; dry; leathery; or discolored brown, white, or charred. Clotted blood vessels may be seen under the burned skin. Subcutaneous fat may be exposed. Ability for this area to spontaneously reepithelialize is destroyed. The contact burn area (Zone 1) is not painful because superficial nerve endings and blood vessels have been destroyed. However, the surrounding, less severely burned area will be extremely painful. The affected area requires debridement and skin grafting in order to heal.

PRIMARY SURVEY AND RESUSCITATION

Airway

History of being burned in an enclosed space or any signs of respiratory difficulties necessitates evaluation of the airway and definitive management. Inhalation injury may be subtle and signs frequently do not appear in the first 24 hours. Aggressive airway management is required with low threshold to intubate.

Breathing

Breathing can be impaired by the following injuries: direct thermal injury producing upper airway edema and obstruction, inhalation of by-products of combustion, carbon monoxide poisoning, and restricted chest wall motion.

Determine airway patency and breathing effectiveness. Observe the nasopharynx and oropharynx looking for evidence of soot, carbonaceous sputum, irritation of the mucous membranes, and/or increased secretions. Inspect for singed nasal, facial, and eyebrow hairs. Determine the presence of cough, hoarseness, stridor, and gag reflex.

Assume carbon monoxide exposure in patients burned in an enclosed space. Obtain a carboxyhemoglobin level on admission. Progressively increased carbon monoxide levels are associated with worsening clinical signs and symptoms (see Table 11-1).

Remember there is increased affinity of carbon monoxide for hemoglobin, which displaces the oxygen from the hemoglobin molecule. Treatment is 100% oxygen via nonrebreather mask or intubation if necessary. Bronchoscopy is highly likely if the patient has inhalation injury, therefore ensure that a large enough endotracheal tube is selected (generally size 7 and above) to accommodate bronchoscopy.

Full-thickness burns of the chest may limit the ability of the chest wall to expand. Gas exchange will be inadequate. If the patient has full-thickness eschar causing respiratory embarrassment then

TABLE 11-1: CARBON MONOXIDE POISONING LEVELS AND SYMPTOMS

CO Level	Symptoms
< 20%	No symptoms
20-30%	Headache and nausea
30-40%	Confusion
40-60%	Coma
> 60	Death

(American College of Surgeons 2004)

escharotomies are required. There will be immediate improvement in the chest wall expansion. Escharotomy is conducted with IV narcotic analgesia. After completion of the procedure, topical antibacterial agents are applied, the limb is elevated, and wet-to-dry gauze dressings are applied.

Circulation

Hypovolemia in the burn patient occurs due to fluid loss and fluid movement from vasodilation and increased capillary permeability. Manual blood pressure measurements are difficult to obtain and often unreliable. Monitoring hourly urine output is helpful. A Foley urinary catheter should be inserted in patients with burns greater than 20%. Monitor urine output for adequacy based on the patient's weight.

- Adults   0.5 ml / kg / hr

- Child   1.0 ml / kg / hr

- Infant   2.0 ml / kg / hr

Two to four large-bore IV catheters should be placed, preferably not in the leg because of the risk of thrombophlebitis. Peripheral IVs may be inserted into burn tissue if no other access is available, but only as a last resort. Suturing catheters in place may be considered because tape does not hold to burn tissue. Central lines are to be avoided unless used to monitor cardiac pressures.

Lactated Ringer's solution is the preferred IV for burns. It has the added benefit of providing potassium, calcium, and lactate, in addition to the sodium and chloride. It mimics the ions in plasma that are lost with the increased capillary permeability.

Burn patients require 2 to 4 ml of lactated Ringer's solution per kilogram body weight per percent body burn in the first 24 hours to maintain an adequate circulating blood volume and provide adequate urine output (American College of Surgeons, 2004a). Of this amount, one half should be infused in the first 8 hours post burn and the remaining one half should be given over the remaining 16 hours. The calculation should be made from the time of the actual burn, not arrival to the hospital.

In full-thickness injuries or those patients with pulmonary injury, fluid requirements are increased. It is necessary to administer the higher resuscitation volume (4 ml/kg) and assess the response frequently.

There is no standard formula for calculating fluid resuscitation in patients with electrical injuries. It is important to increase the urine output in order to excrete myoglobin. Urine outputs as high as 100 ml/hr are sought in electrical injuries. Mannitol may also be given to increase urine flow once urine output is confirmed. Caution should be taken with this formula, as it is only an estimate of fluid need. The volume of IV fluid given should be carefully adjusted according to the individual patient's response as monitored by urinary output, vital signs, and general overall condition.

CASE STUDY

A 70 kg 40-year-old female sustains full-thickness, deep partial-thickness burns to her entire right leg circumferentially, her anterior torso, and her anterior right forearm and hand at 6 a.m. in a house fire.

Questions:

1. Estimate the extent of her burns using the Rule of Nines.

2. Calculate the fluid requirements for:

   a. The first 24 hours postburn

   b. The first 8 hours postburn

Answers:

1. Burn extent using Rule of Nines:

Entire right leg	=	18.0%
Anterior torso	=	18.0%
Anterior forearm	=	4.5%
		40.5%

2. Calculate the fluid requirements for:

   a. the first 24 hours postburn
      (70 x 40 x 4 = 11,200 ml)

   b. the first 8 hours postburn
      (11,200/2 = 5,600 ml)

Temperature Regulation

Skin is the main organ for regulation of body temperature. A burn can disrupt or destroy this function. Further heat loss can occur from the flushing of burned tissue, administration of IV fluids, and the cool environment of the emergency department.

Keep heat loss at a minimum by covering the patient with warm blankets, using warmed IV fluids, warmed humidified air for the ventilator circuit, head covering, increasing the room temperature, and using an overhead warmer.

Wound Care

1. Remove all of the patient's jewelry

2. Assess the status of distal circulation. Use of a Doppler ultrasonic flow meter may be necessary to assess the peripheral pulses.

3. Apply clean white sheets and warm blankets over the wounds. The priority is not the wound, but the respiratory and hemodynamic stability of the patient. Superficial burns are painful but do not require any special wound care. Topical or oral analgesics may be used.

4. Apply a topical antimicrobial agent, such as Silvadene,® Sulfamylon,® silver nitrate solution, gentamicin, and bacitracin; excision and pri-

mary closure; and excision and grafting depending on the burn.

5. Clean the patient's burns with tap water in a shower, bathtub, or tank using clean cloths and coarse wet-to-dry gauze dressings.

6. Break and remove blisters larger than a half-dollar, except on the hands and soles of the feet.

7. Hair should be shaved from burns and nearby areas, followed by covering with topical antibiotic ointment, such as Silvadene® or bacitracin.

8. Irrigate chemical burns immediately with tap water or saline solution for at least 10 min, or until the chemical is completely removed from the skin. Include irrigating areas adjacent to the burns, as they may be injured but will not show signs of pain, blistering, or erythema. After complete flushing, treat the same as a thermal burn.

9. Irrigate eye injuries thoroughly with copious amounts of water or saline solution. Obtain an ophthalmology consult immediately.

10. Apply mineral oil or petroleum jelly to tar or asphalt injuries. Immediately cool with ice, which will loosen the tar allowing you to remove the substance from the injured tissue.

11. Clean electrical wounds gently with water or saline solution. Electrical injuries may have muscle injury but little external tissue loss. However, electrical burns can be extremely deep and serious. The extremities can have considerable damage and tissue swelling, putting the patient at risk for compartment syndrome, which is indicated by pain, pallor, paresthesia, pulselessness, and paralysis. Use extreme care handling the limbs, as the large vessels can tear, leading to massive hemorrhage.

Gastric Tube Insertion

Insert a nasogastric tube and attach it to suction. Patients with more then 20% burn often suffer from an ileus and can vomit and aspirate.

Narcotics, Analgesics, and Sedatives

Narcotics, analgesics, and sedatives should be administered in small frequent doses by the IV routes only.

Criteria for Transfer

The American Burn Association has identified the following types of burns that require transfer to a burn center (American College of Surgeons, 2004a):

1. Partial-thickness and full-thickness burns greater than 10% of the total BSA in patients younger than age 10 or over age 50.

2. Partial-thickness and full-thickness burns greater than 20% BSA in other age-groups.

3. Partial-thickness and full-thickness burns involving the face, eyes, ears, hands, feet, genitalia, or perineum or those that involve skin overlying major joints.

4. Full-thickness burns greater than 5% BSA in any age-group.

5. Significant electrical burns, including lightning injury.

6. Significant chemical burns.

7. Inhalation injury.

8. Burn injury in patients with preexisting illness that could complicate management, prolong recovery, or affect mortality.

COLD INJURY

Cold injury depends on temperature, duration of exposure, environmental conditions, amount of protective clothing, and the patient's general state of health.

Frostnip

Frostnip is the mildest form of cold injury. Signs and symptoms include pain, pallor, and numbness of the body part. It is easily reversible with rewarming and does not result in any tissue loss.

Frostbite

Frostbite is due to freezing tissue. When rewarmed there may be even further injury. Frostbite can be classified as superficial or deep.

Trench Foot or Cold Immersion

This injury is a nonfreezing of the hands or feet, typically seen in soldiers, sailors, or fisherman resulting from chronic exposure to wet conditions and temperatures just above freezing.

Treatment of Cold Injuries

Treatment should be immediate to decrease the time of tissue freezing.

- Ensure adequate ABCs of resuscitation.
- Remove constricting and damp clothing.
- Monitor patient's core temperature.
- Cover with warm blankets.
- Administer hot fluids orally.
- Place the injured body part in circulating warm water.
- Avoid dry heat.
- Do not rub or massage the injured area.

HYPOTHERMIA

Hypothermia is defined as core temperature below 95° F (35° C). Hypothermia can be a solitary event, due to environmental exposure, or it may be associated with trauma. Any degree of hypothermia in trauma patients is considered detrimental.

Treatment of Hypothermia

- Remove the patient from the cold environment. Remove wet, cold clothing, and cover with warm blankets.
- Administer warm oxygen.
- Administer warmed IV fluids to 76° F (42° C).
- Initiate cardiac monitoring.
- Raise temperature to 95° F (35° C) before pro-

nouncing the patient dead. Remember the axiom, you are not dead until you are warm and dead.

SUMMARY

Burns are potentially the most painful and serious injuries that a person can sustain. They are defined as occurring when the body receives more energy than it can absorb without damage.

Burns have a variety of causes: thermal, including scalds, flame, flash, and contact; light; electrical, including shock and lightning; chemical, including contact and inhalation; nuclear; and cold injuries, such as frostbite.

The seriousness of the burn is determined by five factors: evaluation of the burn's depth and damage, extent of injury, involvement of critical areas, patient's age, and the patient's general health and current injury status.

Associated injuries are common, including falls from a height, fractures, and violent muscle contractions. Infections are a high risk with open wounds and foreign bodies. Pulmonary disorders from inhalation damage lead to many deaths. Disfigurement from burns can be grotesque and change or destroy the quality of the patient's life.

Careful history and noting physical findings, as well as measuring temperature, diagnose cold injury. Rewarming techniques should be employed along with frequent vital sign monitoring.

EXAM QUESTIONS

CHAPTER 11

Questions 67-71

67. The skin

    a. is the largest membrane in the body.

    b. functions as the main regulator of the body's balance.

    c. protects the body from bacteria because of it's filter-like qualities.

    d. helps to maintain body temperature through evaporation of sweat.

68. Pulmonary response to smoke inhalation

    a. causes bronchial asthma.

    b. causes carbon monoxide intoxication, upper airway obstruction, and chemical damage to lower airways.

    c. is easily cleared with 100% oxygen administration.

    d. is only a problem in the elderly patient.

69. A patient who has been in an industrial explosion is brought into the emergency department. He is burned on his entire front torso, both circumferential legs, and genitals. What percent TBSA has been burned?

    a. 36%

    b. 45%

    c. 55%

    d. 60%

70. A 13-year-old girl is involved in a garage explosion. She arrives to the emergency department with singed eyebrows, and 25% partial-thickness burns to her face, arms, chest, and hands. She is hoarse and tachypneic. The first management priority is to

    a. start IVs.

    b. administer morphine.

    c. intubate the patient.

    d. debride the wound.

71. The initial treatment for frostbite includes

    a. warm water bath.

    b. vasodilators.

    c. topical application of silvadene.

    d. padding and elevation.

CHAPTER 12

PREGNANCY TRAUMA

CHAPTER OBJECTIVE

Upon completion of this chapter, the reader will be able to describe the principles of treating trauma in pregnancy.

LEARNING OBJECTIVES

Upon completion of this chapter, the reader should be able to

1. recognize normal changes in anatomy and physiology during pregnancy.

2. identify common mechanisms of injury in trauma in pregnancy.

3. identify frequent injuries seen in trauma in pregnancy.

4. describe appropriate nursing assessment of the pregnant trauma patient.

5. choose appropriate interventions for the pregnant trauma patient.

INTRODUCTION

Trauma is the leading cause of death in women during the reproductive years. Trauma during pregnancy involves the safety and lives of both the mother and child. The number one cause of fetal death in trauma is maternal death. The fetal outcome is directly correlated to the mother's outcome. Specific data on the incidence of obstetric trauma is vague, but it is estimated to occur in only about 6% to 7% of pregnant women.

CHANGES IN ANATOMY AND PHYSIOLOGY DURING PREGNANCY

Terminology

Amniotic Sac: A thin, transparent sac, which is the part of the fetal membrane in the uterus that holds the fetus and the fluid in which the fetus is suspended (see Figure 12-1). At the end of the third month of pregnancy, the amnion fuses with the chorion to form the amniochorionic sac. Another term is the "bag of waters."

Amniotic Fluid: The fluid is in the amniotic sac that surrounds the fetus. Transparent, the liquid protects the fetus from injury, maintains an even temperature, and prevents the formation of adhesions between the amnion and the skin of the fetus.

Embryo: The stage in prenatal development between being an ovum and a fetus, from the 2nd to the 8th weeks of gestation.

Fetus: The developing child in utero from the 3rd month to birth.

Gestation: The period of time from conception to birth. The length of pregnancy is normally 38-40 weeks. Fetuses have survived as early as 24-26 weeks of gestation.

FIGURE 12-1: THE STRUCTURE OF PREGNANCY

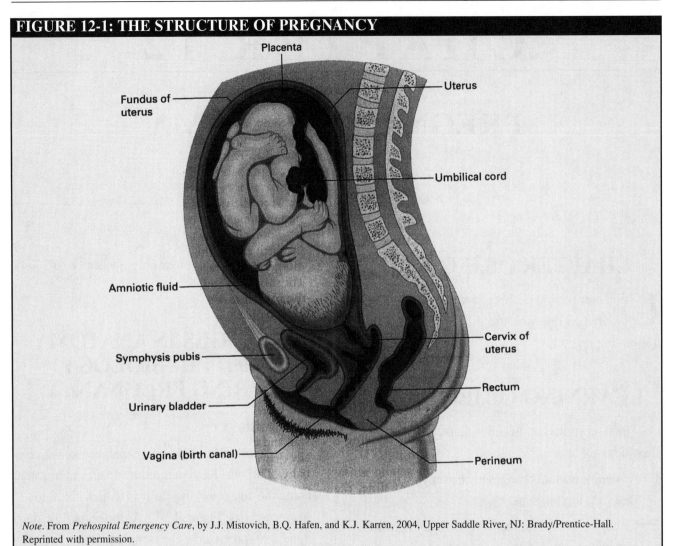

Note. From *Prehospital Emergency Care*, by J.J. Mistovich, B.Q. Hafen, and K.J. Karren, 2004, Upper Saddle River, NJ: Brady/Prentice-Hall. Reprinted with permission.

Gravid: Pregnant

Ovum: The female germ cell capable of developing into a new organism after being fertilized. The egg.

Placenta: A spongy structure in the uterus through which the fetus is nourished. The amnion encloses the embryo and is attached to the margin of the placenta. The umbilical cord is attached at the center of the concave side. Two arteries and one vein comprise the umbilical vessels that pass through the cord. At birth, the cord can be 20 in. (50 cm) in length. After the birth, the placenta is expelled and is called the afterbirth. Maternal blood enters the placenta through branches of the uterine arteries. Nourishment, oxygen, and antibodies from the mother pass into the fetal blood; metabolic waste products pass from fetal blood into the mother's blood. There is no direct mixture of the fetal and maternal blood. The placenta also functions as an endocrine organ, producing gonadotropins (which, if present in urine, is one way to determine pregnancy), estrogen, and progesterone.

Umbilical Cord: The cord connects the fetus with the placenta and contains two arteries and one vein and is surrounded by a jelly-like substance, Wharton's jelly. After the child is born and after the umbilical vessels have stopped pulsating, the umbilical cord is severed. When the stump of the cord dries and falls off, it leaves a depression in the abdomen called the navel or umbilicus.

Structures, Organs, and Systems

Uterus

The uterus is shaped like a pear and expands as the fetus grows. During the first trimester, the uterus is small, self-contained and protected within the pelvis. As the uterus grows, the walls become thinner as it expands outward and upward, pushing on the peritoneal cavity and confining the intestines to the upper abdomen.

In the second trimester, the uterus becomes more susceptible to abdominal injury. The fetus still remains small and well cushioned by the amniotic fluid.

The uterus is large and thin walled by the third trimester. In the last 2 weeks of gestation, the fetus descends and the head becomes "engaged," or fixed in the pelvis, preparing for birth.

Blood flow in the uterus increases from 60 ml/min to 600 ml/min during the third trimester. Total maternal blood volume circulates through the uterus approximately every 8 to 11 minutes. Uterine blood flow is not automatically regulated, and depends completely on the perfusion pressure of the mother. By the third trimester, the uterus and placenta have reached the maximum ability for vasodilation and cannot increase blood flow any further in response to decreased perfusion. Uterine trauma may be a cause of major blood loss.

If there is maternal stress or injury, the sympathetic nervous system releases catecholamines that cause uteroplacental constriction and decreased perfusion. Fetal distress is the consequence.

Cardiovascular

The physiology of the heart changes considerably during pregnancy. The needs of the fetus and mother are highly demanding. Maternal plasma flow increases 40 to 50% by the 28th week. Further, during vaginal delivery, blood loss is about 500 ml, and 1 L during a cesarean delivery.

In the first trimester, systolic and diastolic pressures decrease and then level off in the second trimester. The resting heart rate increases until the second trimester and stays elevated 10 to 20 beats. Complications of pregnancy, such as preeclampsia, will cause a rise in the blood pressure, which may become critical.

Caution: Hypertension in the pregnant patient may indicate an obstetrical complication.

Cardiovascular Changes in Pregnancy:

- Increased pulse

- Increased stroke volume and cardiac output

- Decreased blood pressure

The uterus pushes up the diaphragm so that it elevates the heart and rotates it forward. The shift in position can cause cardiac electrical changes, which are expected in pregnancy.

After 20 weeks' gestation, when the mother is lying down, the fetus may compress the aorta and vena cava, decreasing cardiac output. Compression of the vena cava may decrease the cardiac output by as much as 28% and the systolic blood pressure by 30 mm Hg (Moore et al., 2004). Because blood flow in the uterus is controlled by the maternal perfusion pressure, the changes can decrease perfusion in the uterus. At a time when uterine vasodilation is expanded to the maximum point, the vessels are unable to respond any further to the demand for increased blood flow.

- Position the mother on her left side (left lateral decubitus position) or tilt the backboard toward the left side at a 20-degree angle.

In maternal shock with hypovolemia there will be a compensatory inhibition of vagal tone and release of catecholamines. The effect of this response is to produce vasoconstriction and tachycardia. This vasoconstriction profoundly affects the uterus causing fetal hypoxia and distress. Uterine vasoconstriction leads to reduction in uterine blood flow by 20-30%.

CAUTION:

- The pregnant trauma patient can lose up to 1,500 cc of blood before any detectable change is noted in the blood pressure of the mother. (Campbell, 2004.)

- Pregnant women in shock do not always have the physical indicators of cool, clammy skin, due to vasodilation in the first two trimesters.

- The fetus is compromised with a maternal blood loss of 15-30%.

- The fetus may be in distress despite a stable mother.

- The fetus is often the first to show evidence of decreased uterine perfusion therefore assess fetus for:

  — Changes in fetal movement

  — Fetal tachycardia or bradycardia (normal fetal heart rate is 120-160 beats/min

Pulmonary

Table 12-1 describes significant changes in the pulmonary system that occur during pregnancy. These include an increase in the amount of air moving in and out of lungs with each breath (tidal volume), an increase in the maximum amount of air exhaled from point of maximum inspiration (vital capacity), an increase in respiratory rate with arterial blood gas levels reflecting hyperventilation and compensated respiratory alkalosis, and a decrease in the volume of air in the lungs at end expiration (functional residual capacity) due to elevated diaphragm.

TABLE 12-1: PULMONARY SYSTEM CHANGES DURING PREGNANCY
Increased tidal volume
Increased vital capacity
Increased respiratory rate
Decreased functional residual capacity

Elevation of the diaphragm reduces the mother's pulmonary functional reserve capacity. The capacity is also reduced because of increased maternal oxygen consumption. The diminished functional oxygen reserve in the mother makes the uterus susceptible to hypoxia, which affects fetal oxygenation. When fetal respiratory compromise occurs, the first sign is often a change in the fetal heart rate. In the case of maternal trauma, blood gas levels should be monitored to determine if hypoxia and acidosis have occurred. Supplemental oxygen at 100% is required.

Neurologic

The nervous system does not normally have physiological changes during gestation. Changes in the central nervous system (CNS) during pregnancy may be indicative of pregnancy-induced hypertension (PIH), which may cause seizures and symptoms similar to a head injury.

Pregnancy-Induced Hypertension (PIH)

PIH, also known as toxemia, includes preeclampsia and eclampsia. It is a syndrome occurring between the 20th week and the end of the first week postpartum, and usually is seen in primigravida women younger than age 20 or over age 35. Indications of preeclampsia are hypertension, headaches, proteinuria, decreased urinary output, and edema of the lower extremities. If left untreated, CNS irritability can lead to eclampsia, which magnifies and worsens preeclamptic symptoms and leads to seizure activity. Seizures can cause hypoxia, placing the mother and fetus at risk. Coma may also occur, and pulmonary edema may develop. The condition is an immediate threat to mother and fetus and a leading cause of maternal morbidity and mortality.

Head injury can cause altered mental status, seizures, and hypertension. Careful neurologic assessment is essential in the pregnant trauma patient.

Endocrine

The pituitary gland will double in size and weight and need an increased blood supply by the end of the pregnancy. Low perfusion will bring about ischemia and may lead to pituitary necrosis.

Sheehan's syndrome is necrosis of the anterior pituitary and has long-term complications related to decreased hormone levels.

Shock from hypoperfusion should have rapid and aggressive treatment to prevent ischemia and necrosis. Reperfusion can bring about intrapituitary hemorrhage; carefully monitor the patient.

Gastrointestinal

Several anatomic and physiologic changes occur during gestation. The small bowel is pushed into the upper abdomen by the uterus. The large bowel moves posteriorly. Bowel sounds may be diminished as a normal condition or may be a sign of intraperitoneal injury. Progesterone affects the gastrointestinal tract by reducing motility and tone while relaxing the gastric sphincter. Early insertion of a nasogastric (NG) tube is necessary to minimize the risk of aspiration. The mucosal lining of the respiratory tract is engorged and susceptible to nosebleeds. Extra care should be taken while the NG tube is being inserted.

As the abdominal wall stretches, it becomes less sensitive to peritoneal irritation, causing muscle guarding, rigidity, or rebound tenderness to be dulled or absent, making abdominal physical examination difficult.

Genitourinary

By the end of the first trimester, the bladder moves from a pelvic position to an intra-abdominal position, making it more vulnerable to injury.

The uterus compresses the bladder by the third trimester, causing urinary frequency. Urinary stasis may occur from dilation of the ureters, due to compression by the ovarian plexus.

The filtration rate of the kidneys increases by about 30%. Glycosuria is common, yet proteinuria is not.

Musculoskeletal

As the pelvis prepares for pregnancy, it becomes more flexible. Hormonal changes loosen the ligaments of the symphysis pubis and sacroiliac joints. There is significant widening of the symphysis pubis by the seventh month. Because of these changes, the pelvis is less susceptible to fractures.

Hematology

The increase in plasma volume is much greater than the increase in erythrocyte volume, which causes dilutional anemia. Hematocrit drops because of the red blood cell dilution in the plasma volume. This is referred to as the physiological anemia of pregnancy.

Platelet levels may stay the same or decrease slightly. By term the white count and sedimentation rate have elevated. Fibrinogen levels rise, causing an increased tendency to clot and a risk of deep vein thrombosis or pulmonary embolism. The injured pregnant patient is predisposed to disseminated intravascular coagulation if placental abruption or amniotic fluid embolus occurs.

Laboratory Value Changes in Pregnancy

- Decreased hematocrit
- Increased white blood count
- Increased fibrinogen

MECHANISM OF INJURY

Obviously, trauma can affect both the mother and child. Risks vary according to the stage of gestation and the changing vulnerability of the uterus. However, the stability of the mother most often predicts the outcome of the fetus.

In the first trimester, the fetus has little chance of direct injury because the uterus is still small and protected by the pelvis. However, if the mother is injured, the fetus may suffer consequences from her injuries, such as hypoxia and decreased perfusion. By the last trimester, the uterus and fetus are more likely to be injured from direct trauma because of the expanded anatomical position.

The most common causes of abdominal trauma are motor vehicle crashes, falls, and assaults. Other sources of injury are penetration, domestic violence, burns, and smoke inhalation.

As in any case of blunt trauma, the severity of injury ranges from minor to life-threatening to the mother and fetus. Blunt abdominal trauma from rapid forward deceleration such as car crashes, directs the energy through the abdomen, compressing the organs and structures against the spine. The fetus often takes the direct hit in trauma to the abdomen. In the third trimester, when the uterus is high in the abdomen and the fetus is exposed, the transferred energy can be a deadly force. The uterus may rupture or the placenta may separate from the wall of the uterus. Massive hemorrhage and death of the mother and fetus can result. If the force is great enough to fracture the pelvis of the mother, the fetal skull may also be fractured.

Seat Belt Use

If worn correctly seat belts do not cause harm to the mother or baby. The lap belt should be positioned across the anterior iliac crests of the pelvis and low under the protruding abdomen. Choosing not to wear a seat belt based on the erroneous idea it might injure the fetus only contributes to the possibility of injury. Ejection from the vehicle is more likely to occur when a shoulder harness and/or lap restraint is not used. The mother is apt to have head trauma when ejected and fetal fatality is more likely to happen. Seat belts can cause serious injury, but the risks to mother and fetus are greater without them. Air bag use has also been shown to be safe for the mother and fetus.

The potential for a fall increases because hormonal changes soften joints and relax the pelvic ligaments. As a result, the mother has unstable balance and gait, a protruding abdomen, and she is easily tired. All of these factors make her more susceptible to a fall. Most falls happen during the third trimester.

Gunshots and stab wounds are the predominant cause of penetrating trauma. The probability of fetal injury is related to the point of contact of the penetrating mechanism, the stage of pregnancy, and fetal position. Uterine growth displacing the stomach and small intestines provides some protection for the mother against penetrating trauma. Although multiple organ injury to the mother is less likely to occur, the fetus is often wounded. Fetal mortality rate in penetrating trauma is 70%.

Domestic Violence

Physical abuse among women is increasing, and is often exacerbated during pregnancy. It occurs regardless of ethnic background, cultural influences, or socioeconomic status.

Factors that may "suggest" the presence of domestic violence include:

- Injuries inconsistent with stated history

- Diminished self-image, depression

- Self-abuse

- Frequent emergency department or physician office visits

- Self-blame for injuries

SELECTED OBSTETRIC INJURIES

Premature Labor

The most frequent obstetric trauma complication is the onset of premature labor. Damaged cells release prostaglandin, a chemical that begins contractions. Basically, the degree of uterine damage, fetal age, and amount of prostaglandin released determine the progression of the contractions and labor. Premature labor usually can be detected in alert patients. However in unconscious or intubated patient it can be easily missed. Generally, the contractions are self-limiting, and medical suppression is not necessary. If the contractions proceed, it may indicate other uterine complications such as abruptio placenta. Tocolysis, pharmacological suppression of contractions, may be effective in abating the contractions. Appropriate fluid replacement and positioning the mother in the left lateral tilt position will minimize the uterine irritability.

Signs and Symptoms:

- Uterine contractions greater than 6/hr
- Back pain
- Cervical dilation or effacement

Abruptio Placenta

The most common cause of fetal death after blunt maternal injury is due to separation of the placenta from the uterus. Rarely, minor injury will cause abruption. Abruptio placenta is the leading cause of fetal death not related to maternal death. If the degree of separation exceeds 50%, then the fetal mortality approaches 100% (Moore et al., 2004). Because all gas exchange between the mother and the fetus is across the placenta, the oxygen to the fetus decreases in abruptio while the carbon dioxide increases in the fetal circulation. Fetal insult or death may occur and is related to the time between the separation of the placenta and delivery of the infant.

Signs and Symptoms:

- Vaginal bleeding (may be present or absent)
- Uterine tenderness
- Abdominal pain
- Maternal shock
- Increasing fundal height and fetal distress
- Fetal distress (fetal monitoring should continue until the obstetrician states otherwise). Fetal distress requires immediate surgery. It is possible for the fetus to survive a small abruption.

Uterine Rupture

A direct blow to the abdomen or extreme compression injury can cause a rupture of the uterus. Previous cesarean section is vulnerable at the suture line, making it a predisposing factor. Although rare, it is highly lethal to the fetus and is usually associated with severe maternal injuries. Uterine rupture may be associated with pelvic fractures and bladder rupture. The clinical presentation is often dramatic with severe abdominal pain and distention, palpable fetal parts, and shock. Maternal death generally is associated with additional injuries and happens in less than 10% of the time whereas fetal death is close to 100%. The uterus usually cannot be repaired and a hysterectomy is indicated.

Signs and Symptoms:

- Abdominal pain
- Uterine tenderness
- Absent fetal heart tones
- Change in fundal height or abnormal contour of uterus
- Vaginal bleeding
- Maternal shock

Perimortem Cesarean Section

In rare circumstances, there has been successful emergency cesarean section with deliver of a viable fetus in pregnant trauma victims in cardiopulmonary arrest. The timing is critical and the section should be performed within 5-10 minutes of witnessed arrest.

- Immediately assess gestational age for viability (greater than or equal to 24-26 weeks)
- Prompt CPR initiation at first signs of maternal arrest
- Availability of neonatal resuscitation team

ASSESSMENT

History

Questions to ask:

- What was the mechanism of injury?
- Was the patient wearing a seat belt?
- When was the last menstrual period?
- When is the expected date of confinement (EDC)?
- Have there been any complications during this pregnancy?
- Is there fetal activity? Does the mother feel the fetus moving?

- Are there any uterine contractions or abdominal pain?

Initial Assessment and Treatment

Initial assessment priorities for an injured pregnant patient remain the same as for the nonpregnant patient. As with any trauma patient, the first priorities are the ABCs.

- Assure patent airway, adequate ventilation, and oxygenation.

- Logroll patient toward her left side (tilt backboard 15 to 20 degrees to the left) or manually displace uterus to the left side with a roll under right flank.

- Administer lactated Ringer's solution or normal saline solution IV fluid via two large-bore catheters.

- Avoid administration of vasopressors for the hypotensive pregnant trauma patient.

- Administer type specific blood when at all possible. For hemodynamically unstable bleeding patients the use of emergency uncrossmatched type O Rh negative blood is preferred.

- Insert NG tube early to prevent aspiration.

- Insert Foley catheter to monitor urine output.

- Inspect the perineum.

- Determine if there is any vaginal bleeding or presence of amniotic fluid.

- A pH of 7 to 7.5 in the vagina suggests the presence of amniotic fluid, which indicates ruptured membranes.

- Inspect the vaginal opening for crowning.

- Observe shape and contour of abdomen.

- Auscultate fetal heart tones and rate.

  — Initial fetal heart tones can be auscultated with a Doppler (at 10 weeks or greater gestation).

  — Normal fetal heart tones (FHT) are 120-160 beats /min.

  — Bradycardia is a sustained fetal heart rate less than 110.

  — Tachycardic is a sustained fetal heart rate greater then 160.

- Palpate fundal height to estimate gestational age. The fundus is measured in cm from the symphysis pubis to the top of the fundus. The fundus can usually be palpated by 12 to 14 weeks gestation, and it reaches the umbilicus by 20 weeks. When the fundus is just below the xiphoid, the fetus is full term.

- Palpate the uterus for uterine tenderness or contractions.

- Indications for focused assessment sonography in trauma (FAST) examination, Diagnostic Peritoneal Lavage (DPL), or abdominal computed tomography scan are the same as in the nonpregnant patient. If a DPL is performed, the catheter should be placed above the umbilicus using an open technique. Shield the uterus for all necessary radiographs and avoid all duplication of films.

- Perform a fetal ultrasound to detect fetal cardiac activity, movement, location, approximate age and the amount of amniotic fluid. Fetal death can also be confirmed.

- Initiate fetal heart rate (FHR) monitoring as soon as possible but avoid interference with maternal resuscitation and stabilization. Continuous fetal heart rate monitoring is required for patients with a gestational age of at least 20 to 24 weeks gestation for a minimum of 4 to 6 hours.

  — Ensure that qualified personnel responsible for FHR monitoring are always available.

- Obtain early obstetric consult.

- Kleihauer-Betke Test

  — This test determines whether fetal red cells are in the maternal circulation indicating hemorrhage of fetal blood through the placenta into the mother's circulation. This test is especially important for women who are Rh negative and have a fetus that is Rh positive.

— All pregnant Rh-negative trauma patients should be considered for Rh immunoglobulin therapy unless the injury is very distant from the abdomen. Therapy should be instituted within 72 hours of injury and is determined by the obstetrician.

SUMMARY

Remember the initial management of the pregnant trauma patient is directed at resuscitation and stabilization. The fetus is totally dependent on the mother's well being. The number one cause of fetal demise is maternal demise. Fetal monitoring should be maintained after satisfactory resuscitation and stabilization of the mother. It is important that the trauma surgeon work together with the obstetrician for the best outcome of the two patients.

EXAM QUESTIONS

CHAPTER 12

Questions 72-77

72. Which of the following changes best characterizes the normal response to pregnancy in the third trimester?

   a. Decrease in plasma volume

   b. Decrease in cardiac output

   c. Decrease in tidal volume

   d. Widening of the symphysis pubis

73. Which of the following best characterizes the pregnant trauma patient's response to increased catecholamine release in shock?

   a. Increased maternal renal blood flow

   b. Fetal/maternal dysrhythmias

   c. Improved uterine blood flow

   d. Fetal hypoxia and distress

74. Which of the following best characterizes mechanisms and patterns of injury in pregnant trauma?

   a. The uterus is more vulnerable to injury in the first trimester.

   b. Rapid deceleration in an MVC results in a stalled delivery process.

   c. Maternal pelvic fractures are associated with fetal skull fractures.

   d. Assault is the most frequent mechanism of injury in pregnant females.

75. The most important factor that determines fetal outcome following trauma during pregnancy is

   a. the stability of the mother.

   b. history of blunt abdominal trauma.

   c. degree of fetomaternal hemorrhage.

   d. gestational age or maturity of the fetus.

76. The most common cause of fetal death after blunt injury to a pregnant woman is

   a. ruptured uterus.

   b. prolapsed cord.

   c. abruptio placenta.

   d. premature labor.

77. A pregnant trauma patient should be transported in which position?

   a. Back with head elevated

   b. Back with feet elevated

   c. Right side

   d. Left side

CHAPTER 13

PEDIATRIC TRAUMA

CHAPTER OBJECTIVE

Upon completion of this chapter, the reader will be able to identify the important strategies in management of pediatric patients suffering traumatic injuries.

LEARNING OBJECTIVES

Upon completion of this chapter, the reader should be able to

1. identify the unique characteristics of a child's anatomy and physiology.

2. describe the common mechanisms of injury seen in pediatric trauma.

3. identify common pediatric trauma injuries.

4. specify appropriate assessment of a pediatric trauma patient.

5. select appropriate nursing interventions for the pediatric trauma patient.

INTRODUCTION

It is often said in the field of pediatrics that children are not little adults. This is true. Children do have unique anatomic and physiologic characteristics. There are biophysical, psychosocial, and cognitive differences that distinguish them from adults. However, priorities for the initial treatment is the same for children as it is for adults.

Trauma morbidity and mortality exceed all major diseases in children and young adults, making injury the most serious public health and health care problem in this population.

FINANCIAL BURDEN OF PEDIATRIC TRAUMA

Pediatric trauma care is more costly than trauma care for adults, including hospitalization, resources for rehabilitation, mainstreaming the child back into society, and the years of potential work loss. Medical expenses are in the billions of dollars, not to mention the costs to society. Prevention is less expensive and more beneficial.

ANATOMY AND PHYSICAL CHARACTERISTICS OF CHILDREN

Physical Growth

The first year of life sees tremendous changes in growth and development. Average birth weight doubles in 6 months and triples by the end of the year. After that time, weight gain slows to about 2.5 kg (1 kg equals 2.2 lb) a year during the preschool and school years.

The child has a higher center of gravity. The infant's head is large in relation to his or her body, allowing a significant amount of heat to be lost through the scalp. The combination of a large head and high center of gravity causes the infant and young child to have poor balance control and be predisposed to falls.

Metabolism and Fluid and Electrolyte Balance

Fluid distribution in infants is different than that of the adult. Seventy-five percent of the infant's weight is water, compared to 60-70% in the adult.

Infants and young children have a metabolic rate 2-3 times greater than older children and adults. Therefore, their caloric, fluid, and oxygen needs are greater. Increased fluid needs and fluid turnover can bring about rapid deficits during periods of decreased fluid intake or increased fluid loss. Dehydration quickly follows.

Thermoregulation

Increased heat loss from the relatively large body surface area-to-weight ratio and the limited ability to produce heat make it difficult for infants and small children to maintain their body temperatures. The large head size accounts for a high percent of surface area and heat loss.

Respiratory System

Newborns normally have adequate pulmonary structures to support oxygenation and ventilation. However, the small airway size and an immature immune system increase the possibility of obstruction and respiratory disorders.

Airway

The neck is short, the tongue is large and trachea is narrower. It takes just a small amount of mucus, a small foreign object, or slight tissue edema to close off the airway (see Figure 13-1).

Infants are nose breathers for the first few months of life and nasal congestion can bring on signs of respiratory distress.

A jaw thrust or chin lift will open the infant or young child's airway.

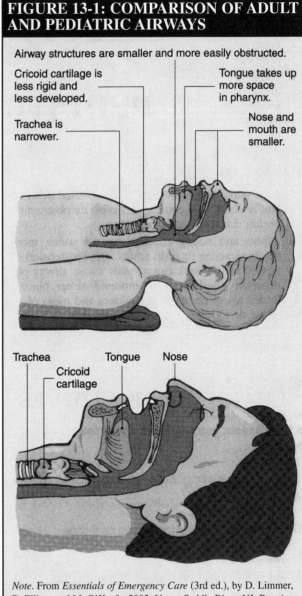

FIGURE 13-1: COMPARISON OF ADULT AND PEDIATRIC AIRWAYS

Airway structures are smaller and more easily obstructed.

Cricoid cartilage is less rigid and less developed.

Tongue takes up more space in pharynx.

Trachea is narrower.

Nose and mouth are smaller.

Trachea

Cricoid cartilage

Tongue

Nose

Note. From *Essentials of Emergency Care* (3rd ed.), by D. Limmer, B. Elling, and M. O'Keefe, 2002, Upper Saddle River, NJ: Prentice Hall. Reprinted with permission.

In children younger than age 8, the cricoid cartilage is the narrowest portion of the trachea. Uncuffed endotracheal tubes are recommended for this age group. The trachea is shorter, increasing the possibility of mainstem intubation.

Breathing

Children younger than age 7 or 8 breathe with their diaphragms or abdomens. The diaphragm is the child's primary muscle of ventilation because the intercostal muscles are poorly developed and contribute little to chest wall movement. In respiratory distress, the diaphragmatic breathing and pliable ribs cause the chest wall to move inward, or retract, during inspiration.

Crying children tend to swallow air, causing gastric distention. The thin chest wall transmits breath sounds easily, making accurate respiratory assessment difficult.

Respiratory rates and oxygen consumption in children is higher because of their faster metabolic rates. Generally the younger the child the faster the respiratory rate (see Table 13-1). Infants and young children have fewer and smaller alveoli than adults, consequently, less pulmonary reserve. Children may become fatigued during the increased work of breathing. Due to diminished respiratory reserve and higher oxygen requirements, untreated respiratory distress can rapidly turn into respiratory failure. The chest wall in infants and young children is more pliable. Blunt trauma to the chest usually results in rib contusions instead of fractures. When there are rib fractures, severe internal trauma is also likely.

Children also have lower glycogen stores but have increased metabolic demands.

Cardiovascular System

The child's normal cardiovascular system has anatomic and physiologic differences from the adult's that affect the child's response to stress.

Blood volume, while actually small in the child, is relatively greater than the adult's. It does not take a great deal of blood loss in the child to impair perfusion and decrease circulating volume. Even with serious blood loss, large cardiac reserve and catecholamine response will maintain a normal blood pressure. **Not until up to 30% of the circulating volume is lost does hypotension become evident.** Hypotension is a late sign of hypovolemia and indicates impending cardiac arrest.

Higher metabolic and oxygen demands in children require higher cardiac output per kilogram. When oxygen decreases, tachycardia is the response. If tachycardia does not increase oxygen

delivery, tissue hypoxia and hypercapnia develop. **Bradycardia follows, which is an ominous sign.**

As a rule, blood pressure increases with the age of the child (see Table 13-1). A neonate usually has a systolic pressure of 50 to 60 mm Hg. The same pressure in a child indicates hypotension. A neonate's heart rate is usually 120 to 160 beats per minute and decreases as the child grows older.

TABLE 13-1: PEDIATRIC VITAL SIGNS BY AGE

Age	Respiratory Rate	Pulse	Blood Pressure
Neonate	40-60	100-180	60-90
Infant	30-60	100-160	87-105
Toddler	24-40	80-110	95-105
Preschooler	22-34	70-110	82-110
School-age	18-30	65-110	97-112
Adolescent	12-16	60-90	112-128

(Limmer, Elling, & O'Keefe, 2002)

Neurologic System

Major neurologic structures are present but incompletely developed at birth. Temperature instability indicates incomplete development of the autonomic system. Infant sensitivity to parasympathetic stimulation is shown by bradycardia with defecation or deep suctioning.

The infant's head is proportionally larger than the adult's. The bones of the cranium are soft and pliable, held together by fibrous sutures to allow for brain growth. This structure allows the skull to cope with increased intracranial pressure (ICP), but it is also less able to protect the brain. The large head and high center of gravity makes a child more prone to falls and head injuries.

Infants can have significant bleeding from a scalp laceration because of the increased vascularity and large surface area.

The cervical spine is vulnerable to injury. The vertebrae will not easily fracture, but the spinal cord is vulnerable.

Musculoskeletal System

Bones are pliable so that greenstick or incomplete fractures are common. The bone growth allows rapid callus formation, which permits bones to heal quickly. Although the bones are strong, fractures happen more frequently than muscle sprains or ligament tears because these structures are stronger than the bones.

The growth, or epiphyseal, plate is unique to children. New longitudinal bone growth is dependent on this cartilaginous area, which does not ossify until puberty. This characteristic allows a fracture to be present without radiographic detection.

Gastrointestinal (GI) and Genitourinary Systems

Undeveloped abdominal muscles are weak and allow children's stomachs to protrude. The small size of a child's abdomen holds the organs close together. These two factors make the abdomen vulnerable to blunt trauma, especially multiple organ injury. Further, pliable ribs not only are inadequate support for the lungs, they do not adequately protect the abdominal organs, which is another factor that places the child at risk for internal injuries.

MECHANISM OF INJURY

Motor vehicle crashes (MVCs) are the leading cause of death in children of all ages, whether the child was a passenger, a pedestrian, or a cyclist. Deaths due to firearms, other transportation (such as off-road, water, and snow vehicles), falls, and drowning follow in descending order (see Figure 13-2) (American College of Surgeons, 2004c). Child abuse accounts for the majority of homicides in infants. Penetrating trauma account for the majority of homicides in children and adolescents (Peiztman et al., 2002). Falls are the second most frequent injury seen, but are the least lethal. Blunt mechanisms of injury and the child's small body often result in multisystem injury much more commonly than isolated injury.

FIGURE 13-2: PEDIATRIC DEATHS BY MECHANISM OF INJURY

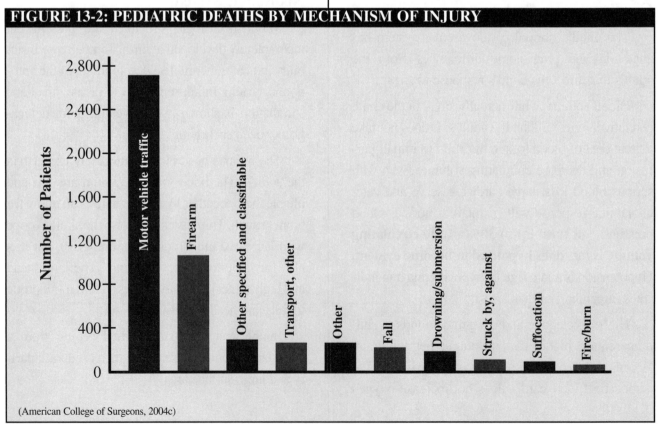

(American College of Surgeons, 2004c)

Motor Vehicle Crashes

Child Safety Seats

It is estimated that up to 70% of youngsters are unrestrained or improperly restrained in vehicles. Car seats have been found to be used only 40% of the time with toddlers (NHTSA, 2002). In a vehicular accident, when unrestrained, young children are thrown around inside the vehicle, they may receive injuries to the head, abdomen, chest, and extremities. They are also at high risk of being thrown through a window. Head injuries are the leading cause of death among unrestrained children. When children are held on the lap of an adult, they can be crushed between the adult and the dashboard or steering column, or against the front seat if they were backseat lap passengers.

Young children can sustain certain seat belt-related injuries due to their body size and proportion. A greater percent of a child's body size is above the safety belt than with an adult, which allows forward motion and an increased chance of head and neck injury. Children can also jackknife over restraints, causing an airway or hanging injury.

Air Bags

Air bags have contributed to serious injuries and deaths of infants and young children because they are deployed when the unrestrained child is thrown against the dashboard during rapid deceleration before impact. Air-bag deployment then propels the child against the structures inside the vehicle. Infants riding in rear-facing safety seats should never ride in the front seat of a car or truck with a passenger-side air bag. All children under age 12 should be restrained in the back seat with a shoulder and lap restraint.

Riding Equipment

All-terrain vehicles, snowmobiles, farm equipment, and riding lawn mowers can be dangerous vehicles and all cause serious injuries and deaths. Whether a young child is riding as a passenger or an older child is operating these vehicles, terrible injuries or death can occur either from carelessness or lack of skill.

Sports

Skateboarding and rollerblading contribute to multiple injuries. Physically, children have a high center of gravity, which interferes with their ability to break a fall. Pediatricians recommend that children under age 5 not use skateboards because they do not have a well-developed neuromuscular system. Additionally, they have poor judgment and are unable to effectively protect themselves from injury. Skateboarders should always wear the proper protective equipment and stay out of traffic.

Pedestrian

Pedestrian injuries in 5- to 9-year-olds are the second greatest killer. Walking, running, crossing a street, and entering or leaving a school bus make up most of the injuries, and occur most often in the afternoon and early evening. When children are struck by a vehicle, a triad of injuries, known as Waddell's triad, occur: thoracic abdominal damage from the bumper, extremity injury from hitting the vehicle and the ground, and head injury from landing on the ground.

Falls

Falls are the most common cause of head injury and trauma-related hospitalization in young and older adults. Young children receive most fall-related injuries in the home due to clutter in the home, infants in walkers, open windows, stairs, climbing, bunk beds, and myriad other situations. For children younger than age 13, falls from a window, and jumping from a bed, stairs, and low heights during rough play are the most common mechanisms of injury.

Child Abuse

Child abuse is associated with head injuries, burns, abdominal injuries, and fractures. One characteristic is an inconsistent story. The stated mechanism of injury often does not match the injury observed. There can often be a significant time lapse between the injury and presentation in the emergency department.

COMMON PEDIATRIC TRAUMA INJURIES

Head Injury

Traumatic brain injury (TBI) is the most common cause of injury-related death in children. Auto crashes and falls cause most head injuries in the pediatric population. Attention to the ABCs is imperative as hypoxia and hypotension from associated injuries can significantly impact the outcome from head injury. Hypotension from hypovolemia is the most significant secondary injury to the brain and should be avoided at all costs.

• In general, children have better outcomes from head injury than adults do.

• Children tend to have fewer focal masses than adults do.

• Children tend to have more brain swelling than adults do.

• Early neurosurgical consultation is imperative.

• Aggressive monitoring of ICP is recommended.

Spinal Cord Injury

Spinal cord injury in children is a relatively rare occurrence. MVCs account for spinal cord injury in children under age 10, whereas MVCs and sporting activities account for spinal cord injury in children over age 10.

More common in children than adults is spinal cord injury without radiographic abnormality (SCIWORA). The pliability of the child's spine will allow cord injury without bony abnormality. Transient displacement of the spinal column is the result of a flexion-extension or acceleration-deceleration force. The head is hyperflexed or hyperextended and the cord stretches, causing injury or transection. This action is followed by the spinal cord returning to its normal length and the verte-

brae realignment. The patient has signs of spinal cord damage, such as paralysis, without radiographic indication.

Thoracic Injury

Most pediatric chest injuries are the result of blunt trauma. In children, energy from blunt force may be transmitted to the internal thoracic structures, the heart, lungs, and great vessels. Because the ribs are undeveloped and flexible, blunt trauma usually causes a contusion rather than a fracture. When a fracture does occur, it is likely the result of considerable force, and there is a good chance of damage to the internal organs. Flail segments should raise suspicion of severe parenchymal injury. Mobility of mediastinal structures makes the child more sensitive to tension pneumothorax and flail segments.

Abdominal Injury

Most pediatric abdominal injuries occur as the result of blunt trauma, primarily involving MVCs and falls.

As with thoracic trauma, blunt force is the most frequent cause of abdominal injury in children. Described before, the abdomen is small with the organs close together, so blunt force is liable to cause damage to more than one organ. In order of frequency of injury is the spleen, liver, pancreas, and intestines. Most of these injuries are handled nonoperatively.

Children restrained only by a lap belt are at risk for a pairing of injuries caused by severe flexion of the spine and the GI tract. As the lap belt-restrained child jackknifes forward in a frontal crash there is a flexion disruption or (Chance) fracture of the lumbar spine. This is frequently seen with an associated small bowel injury. Any patient with this mechanism should be carefully observed for increasing abdominal pain and white blood cell count and have x-rays or computed tomography (CT) scans of the lumbar spine.

Abused Child

The abused child syndrome refers to any child who sustains an intentional injury as the result of caregivers. The terms "child abuse" and "child maltreatment" are used interchangeably to describe neglect and physical, emotional, and sexual abuse. The manner of identifying and reporting maltreatment is directly related to the legal definitions and protocols of the state, city, and hospital. Hospital staff must be well versed in this information and procedures.

Suspected Abuse

- The history and physical injury do not match.

- Significant time interval has passed between the time of injury and seeking help.

- History of repeated trauma and having been treated in different emergency departments.

- Parents respond inappropriately or do not follow medical advice.

- The injury story changes among caregivers.

Clinical Signs Suggestive of Abuse

- Unexplained bruises or welts found on the face, torso, buttocks, back, or thighs, often reflecting the shape of the object used, such as a belt buckle, strap, or fly swatter.

- Unexplained burns on palms, soles of feet, buttocks, or back; burns from a cigarette, electrical appliance; or rope burn.

- Unexplained fractures or dislocations involving the skull, ribs, and bones around joints, including multiple fractures or spiral fractures.

- Other unexplained injuries, such as lacerations, abrasions, a human bite, pinch marks, clumps of lost hair, retinal hemorrhages, or abdominal injuries.

EVALUATION AND MANAGEMENT

Assessment: Primary Survey

Airway

- A patent airway is the starting place in the initial assessment of pediatric trauma.

- **The inability to establish and or maintain a patent airway with lack of oxygenation and ventilation is the MOST COMMON cause of cardiac arrest in the child.**

- To maintain optimal breathing, proper positioning of the child is necessary to avoid passive flexion of the cervical spine caused by a relatively large head.
  - Place the child in neutral position to maintain alignment (see Figure 13-3).
  - Place a layer of padding under the infant or toddler's torso (shoulder to hips) to preserve neutral alignment of the spinal column. This also improves visualization of the vocal cords for intubation.

- Open the airway with the chin lift or jaw thrust maneuver combined with inline spinal immobilization.

- Suction oral airway of secretions or debris.

- Insert oropharyngeal airway in the unconscious child only.
  - Measure the airway from the corner of the mouth to the tip of the earlobe.
  - Avoid the backwards and rotate insertion technique utilized in adults. Trauma to the soft tissues of the child's oropharynx can result.
  - Gently depress the tongue with a tongue blade and insert the oropharyngeal airway directly into the oropharynx.

- Place an orogastric tube to decompress the stomach prior to intubation.
  - Crying children often swallow large amounts of air that can lead to gastric distention, vomiting, and aspiration.

FIGURE 13-3: NEUTRAL POSITIONING OF A CHILD

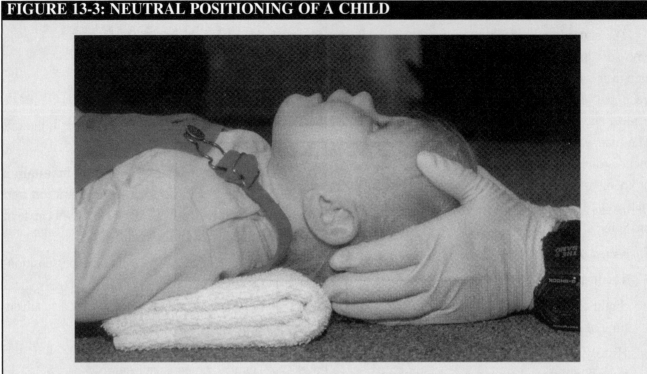

Note. From *Basic Trauma Life Support* by J. Campbell, Ed., 2004, Upper Saddle River, NJ: Prentice Hall. Reprinted with permission.

- Administer supplemental oxygen prior to any intubation attempts.
  - Infants and children have a more pronounced vagal response to endotracheal intubation than adults do. Such responses may be caused by hypoxia or vagal stimulation during laryngoscopy.

- Consider a protocol for emergency intubation referred to as rapid sequence intubation. This protocol while often hospital specific generally consists of the following steps: preoxygenation, atropine to minimize vagal stimulation, etomidate and midazolam for sedation, cricoid pressure to avoid aspiration of gastric contents, and paralysis with short-acting paralytics like succinylcholine prior to intubation.

- Oral intubation is preferred. Nasotracheal intubation is to be avoided.

- Insert uncuffed endotracheal tubes for children younger than 8 years of age.
  - The child's cricoid ring is the narrowest part of the airway and forms a natural seal with the endotracheal tube.

- Determine endotracheal tube size by using the following methods:
  - Match tube size to the diameter of the child's little finger or external nares
  - Use age-based formula:

    Endotracheal tube size (in millimeters) $= \dfrac{\text{Age (yrs)}}{4} + 4$

- Confirm endotracheal tube placement by auscultation of bilateral chest walls in the axillae.
  - The infant's trachea is short, therefore caution is necessary when intubating because the endotracheal tube tends to easily pass into the right mainstem bronchus instead of into the trachea.

- Obtain chest x-ray to verify endotrachial tube placement.

- Recheck breath sounds and tube centimeter depth marking at lip line periodically to ensure that the tube stays in position.
  - Tube placement depth can be estimated by multiplying the diameter of the tube by 3. Example: endotrachial tube diameter size 4 x 3 = 12 cm (lip line)

— Any small movement of the head can cause dislodgement of the tube

- When a surgical airway is required:
  — Needle cricothyroidotomy is preferred in children younger than 12 years of age.
  — Surgical cricothyroidotomy can be performed when the cricothyroid membrane can be palpated usually in children ages 12 and older.

Breathing

- Are respirations spontaneous? What is the respiratory rate?
  — The respiratory rate decreases with age. An infant breathes around 40 to 60 breaths/min, while an older child breathes 20 breaths/min.
- Normal tidal volume varies from 6 to 8 ml/kg for infants and children.
  — Avoid over exertion of manual pressure when bagging as this causes injury to the fragile upper airway tissues and lungs, as well as pushing air into the stomach.

- Assess ventilation by watching the rise and fall of the chest.
  — Remember hypoxia is the most common cause of cardiac arrest in the child. Hypoventilation causes a respiratory acidosis, which can be corrected with adequate ventilation and perfusion.

Circulation

Assessment of shock in children can be subtle and misleading. The increased physiologic reserve of the children allow for maintaining vital signs in a normal range as blood loss occurs. The primary response to hypovolemia is tachycardia (American College of Surgeons, 2004) (see Table 13-2).

- Check apical pulse for rate, rhythm, and quality.
- Check peripheral pulses for quality.
- Place the patient on cardiac monitor.
- Check the patient's skin temperature and color.
- Children are often able to maintain normal vital signs even with shock.
  — Up to 30% of blood loss is required before

TABLE 13-2: SYSTEMIC RESPONSES TO BLOOD LOSS IN PEDIATRIC PATIENTS			
System	**Mild Blood Volume Loss (< 30%)**	**Moderate Blood Volume Loss (30-45%)**	**Severe Blood Volume Loss (> 45%)**
Cardiovascular	Increased heart rate Weak, thready distal pulses	Low normal blood pressure Narrowed pulse pressure Increased heart rate Absent peripheral pulse Thready central pulse	Hypotension Tachycardia Bradycardia
Central Nervous System	Anxious Irritable Confused	Lethargic Dulled response to pain	Comatose
Skin	Cool, mottled Prolonged capillary refill	Cyanotic Markedly prolonged capillary refill	Pale Cold
Urinary	Minimally decreased urine output	Minimal urine output	No urine output

Note. From *Advanced Trauma Life Support for Doctors, Student Course Manual* (7th ed.), by the American College of Surgeons, 2004, Chicago: ACS. Reprinted with permission.

any change will be noted in a child's vital signs.

- Tachycardia and poor skin perfusion are early indicators of hypovolemia.

- Early subtle signs of hypovolemic shock include:
  — Loss of distal peripheral pulses
  — Narrowing of pulse pressure to less than 20 mm Hg
  — Skin mottling
  — Cool extremities compared to trunk with coolness ascending towards the trunk
  — Decrease in level of consciousness
  — Dulled response to pain

- Late sign of hypovolemic shock
  — Decreased blood pressure. Normal systolic blood pressure: SBP = 80 mm Hg + [2 x Age]
  — By the time hypotension is seen in a child greater than 45% of the circulating blood volume is lost
  — Tachycardia often changes to bradycardia at this point

- Venous Access
  — Peripheral IV sites are the preferred route for IV access
  — After two failed attempts within 90 seconds proceed to intraosseous IV insertion
  — Intraosseous IV insertion
    ◆ Preferred sites are proximal tibia below the tibial tuberosity or the distal femur
    ◆ Avoid placing distal to a fracture site
    ◆ Verify placement by aspiration of bone marrow
    ◆ Can be used to infuse fluids, blood, and medication
    ◆ Discontinue as soon as peripheral IV can be established
  — Depending on the skill level available, femoral venous line may also be inserted

- Fluid Resuscitation
  — Administer fluid bolus with warmed lactated Ringer's solution or normal saline solution 20 ml/kg up to 3 times to a total of 60 ml/kg.
  — Consider a bolus of packed red blood cells next (10 ml/kg).
  — Fluid resuscitation based on body weight
  — Many hospitals use the Broselow™ Pediatric Emergency Tape which allows quick estimate of weight, fluid volume, and drug dosages.
  — Continuously monitor the child for improvements in response to fluid administration. Look for the following improvements:
    ◆ Return of peripheral pulses
    ◆ Improved skin color and warmth
    ◆ Slowing pulse rate
    ◆ Improved level of consciousness (LOC)
    ◆ Increased blood pressure
    ◆ Increased urine output
  — If the child does not improve significantly consideration should be given to possible operation.

- Urinary Output
  — Adequate urine output is based on patient's weight
  — Infant = 2 ml/kg/hr
  — Toddler = 1.5 ml/kg/hr
  — Child = 1.0 ml/kg/hr
  — Adolescent = 0.5 ml/kg/hr

- Thermoregulation
  — Children are more sensitive to heat loss due to the high ratio of body surface area to body mass and thin skin and lack of substantial subcutaneous tissue.
  — Use blankets, warmed IV fluids, and ventilator circuits to preserve body temperature.

- Diagnostic Assessment for Bleeding Internal Injury
  - Rapid CT scanning allows for fast, precise identification of injuries.
  - Use of focused assessment sonography in trauma (FAST) is relatively new in pediatric trauma but may be helpful to identify intra-abdominal blood.
  - Diagnostic Peritoneal Lavage (DPL) is used with much less frequency due to the availability of FAST. However, DPL can be used in children when FAST is not available.
- Nonoperative Management
  - Most trauma centers today practice non-operative management of pediatric abdominal injuries.
  - Most bleeding from the spleen, liver, and kidney will generally stop on their own, not requiring surgery.
  - Nonoperative management is carried out under the direction of a surgeon, in a hospital equipped with 24-hour availability of an operating room.

Disability

- Check pupil size.
- Assess LOC using the pediatric Glasgow Coma Scale score, which is adapted by changing the verbal section only (see Table 13-3).

TABLE 13-3: PEDIATRIC GLASGOW COMA SCALE SCORE (VERBAL COMPONENT)

Verbal Response	Verbal Score
Appropriate words or smile	5
Crying but consolable	4
Persistently irritable	3
Restless, agitated	2
No response	1

Expose

- Remove patient's clothing and inspect the entire body.

Secondary Survey

History

Information is gathered on the principle of who, what, where, when, and why the injury occurred. Detailed information is particularly important when the mechanism of injury is a passenger/MVC, pedestrian/MVC, bicycle crash, fall, gunshot or stabbing wound, or there is suspected neglect or abuse. Be sure to find out if the patient had a loss of consciousness, for what duration, and if it was followed by vomiting and visual changes.

Head, Eyes, Ears, and Nose

- Check the scalp for abrasions, lacerations, and open wounds.
- Palpate the scalp for "step-off" defects, depressions, hematomas, and pain.
- Palpate the forehead, orbits, maxilla, and mandible for crepitus, deformities, "step-off" defects, pain, and stability.
- Reassess the pupils; check for extraocular movements; ask the child if he or she has any visual difficulties. Look for raccoon eyes or Battle's sign.
- Note if the ears or nose have rhinorrhea or otorrhea.
- Evaluate for malocclusion by asking the child to open and close his or her mouth; note open wounds and loose, chipped, broken, or missing teeth.
- Check for orthodontic appliances, and note if they are intact.
- Evaluate facial symmetry by asking the child to smile, grimace, and open and close his mouth.
- Do not remove impaled or foreign objects.

Neck

- Carefully open the cervical collar, while another person maintains neck alignment, to reassess the anterior neck for jugular vein distention and tracheal deviation. Note bruising, open wounds, edema, crepitus, debris, or chemicals under the collar.

- Check for hoarseness or changes in the voice by speaking to the child.

Chest

- Note respiratory rate; reassess breath sounds for quality.

- Palpate the chest wall and sternum for pain, tenderness, or crepitus.

- Observe inspiration and expiration for symmetry or paradoxical movement.

- Note use of accessory muscles.

- Reassess apical heart rate, rhythm, and clarity.

Abdomen, Pelvis, Genitourinary

- Look for bruising and distention of the abdomen; auscultate bowel sounds in all four quadrants; palpate the abdomen gently for tenderness; assess the pelvis for tenderness and stability.

- Palpate the bladder for tenderness and distention; check the urinary meatus for injury or bleeding; note priapism, genital trauma, lacerations, or any foreign bodies.

- Confirm rectal sphincter tone and look for lacerations.

Musculoskeletal

- Assess extremities for deformities, swelling, lacerations, or other injuries.

- Palpate distal pulses for presence, quality, rate, and rhythm and compare to central pulses.

- Ask the child to wiggle his or her toes and fingers; evaluate strength of hand grips and foot flexion/extension.

Back

- Logroll the patient, being careful to maintain spinal and neck alignment, to inspect the back; look for bruising and open wounds; palpate all vertebrae for tenderness, pain, deformity, and stability; assess the flank area for bruising and tenderness.

TRANSFER

Children with multisystem injuries can deteriorate rapidly and develop serious complications. Therefore, such patients should be transferred early to a facility capable of managing the child with multisystem injuries. The American College of Surgeons (ACS) suggests that specific centers that treat children should have capabilities above those of a general trauma center. Such centers are recognized by the ACS as trauma centers with a commitment to children or Level I pediatric centers.

SUMMARY

The pediatric patient has unique characteristics and problems for the trauma nurse. Potentially life-threatening injuries must be quickly and accurately identified. Children with multiple injuries, including head injury, must be aggressively resuscitated to avoid any hypotension and secondary brain injury. Early involvement of the general surgeon is necessary to manage the injured child.

EXAM QUESTIONS

CHAPTER 13

Questions 78-85

78. Which of the following statements regarding children and trauma is true?

    a. Children suffer spinal cord injury without x-ray changes.

    b. Children have more focal mass lesions than adults.

    c. Children suffer more spinal cord injuries than adults.

    d. An infant with a closed-head injury may become hypotensive from increased cerebral edema.

79. The number one mechanism of injury resulting in pediatric death is

    a. falls.

    b. sports injury.

    c. gun shot wounds.

    d. MVC.

80. Which of the following best characterize pediatric trauma injuries?

    a. Most pediatric spleen injuries require prompt surgery.

    b. Most pediatric chest injuries result in rib fractures.

    c. Small bowel injuries may occur in children with lap belt injuries.

    d. The most frequent cause of head injury in pediatrics is from child abuse.

81. Up until about age 8, which is the narrowest part of the airway?

    a. Bronchi

    b. Cricoid cartilage

    c. Epiglottis

    d. Larynx

82. A 9-year-old female falls 20 feet from a tree house and is brought into the emergency department by her mother. Her vital signs are normal, but she complains of left upper quadrant pain. An abdominal CT scan reveals a moderately severe laceration of the spleen. The hospital does not have a 24-hour a day operating room capabilities. The most appropriate management of this patient would be to

    a. transfer the patient to a trauma center.

    b. obtain a type and crossmatch for blood.

    c. admit the patient to the Pediatric Intensive Care Unit for careful observation.

    d. prepare the patient for surgery the next day.

83. A 4-year-old boy was a pedestrian struck by a car and brought to the emergency department. His GCS is 3. His BP is 90 mm Hg systolic, heart rate 140 beats/min, and his respiratory rate is 36 breaths/min. The preferred route of venous access in this patient is

    a. intraosseous.

    b. femoral vein.

    c. central venous catheter.

    d. peripheral veins in upper extremity.

84. Which of the following steps best characterizes the positioning of the child's head to optimize breathing?

    a. Raise the head of bed.

    b. Flex the head to prevent airway obstruction.

    c. Place rolled towel under shoulders.

    d. Apply cervical collar to maintain position.

85. Regarding shock, which of the following statements in a child is true?

    a. Hypotension is an early sign of shock.

    b. The pulse rate increases with the age of the patient.

    c. 10 cc/kg/hr is the initial IV bolus used in pediatric resuscitation.

    d. Change in skin temperature and color are early signs of shock.

CHAPTER 14

GERIATRIC TRAUMA

CHAPTER OBJECTIVE

Upon completion of this chapter, the reader will be able to apply the principles of trauma care for managing the acutely injured geriatric patient.

LEARNING OBJECTIVES

Upon completion of this chapter, the reader should be able to

1. identify anatomic and physiologic changes of aging.

2. specify mechanisms of injury common to older adult patients.

3. recognize hallmarks of abuse and neglect seen in the older adult patients.

4. identify the common types of injuries that are seen in older adult patients.

5. choose the interventions appropriate to the management of critical injuries in geriatric patients.

INTRODUCTION

The fastest growing segment of the population is older adults. It is projected that they will represent more than 20% of the U.S. population by the year 2025 (Moore et al., 2004). Older adults are living longer and with better health than ever before. Reasons vary from medical advances to personal awareness of nutrition, fitness, prevention, and care, along with societal support for improved quality of life. Numerous older adults continue to pursue many of the same activities that they did at a much younger age, but at an increased opportunity and risk for injury.

Trauma in the older patient is likely to be more serious than the same injury in the younger person. They develop more complications that are potentially more serious, are hospitalized longer, and have less certain prospects for survival. Although the older adult population (over age 65) represents only 12% of the trauma patients, they make up nearly one third of the trauma-related health care expenditures in this country and account for more than one quarter of the deaths (Moore et al., 2004).

Older adult trauma patients that may appear on initial assessment to have only minor injuries often go on to die. Fully a third of older adult trauma patients that expire, do not actually die from the original injury, but instead succumb to multiple organ failure that so often accompanies injury in older adults (Moore et al., 2004). Unrecognized states of hypoperfusion are thought to be the culprit, which is why early aggressive hemodynamic monitoring is a must in the older adult trauma patient.

Elder abuse and neglect is increasing. There are many reasons, including the increasing aging population and complex problems regarding the caregivers. Abuse is found in all socioeconomic backgrounds and women are more abused than men.

EPIDEMIOLOGY AND MECHANISMS OF INJURY

As stated in the introduction, older adults continue to participate in many of the same activities they did at a younger age because they are in better condition than ever; society now includes them in more activities; and probably, also in defiance of their age. This age group incurs a higher population-based death rate from trauma than any other age group (Moore et al., 2004). The leading causes of death due to injury among older adult patients are falls, motor vehicle crashes (MVC), and burns.

Falls

Falls are the most common cause of injury and death among older adults. Falls represent 40% of the deaths among older adults. The frequency and severity increase with age. Many falls result in an isolated orthopedic injury, such as tripping and fracturing a hip. When an older adult has a fall injury, the cause should be investigated thoroughly. Frequently, falls occur because the aging process causes postural instability, poor balance, alteration in gait, and decreased muscle strength and coordination. Acute or chronic associated conditions such as syncope, cardiac dysrhythmias, hypoglycemia, anemia and transient cerebral ischemia or other gait-altering disorders must also be considered as precipitating factors for falls. For example, an episode of bradycardia may bring on syncope, resulting in a fall. Drugs including alcohol are a common cause or contributing factor to many falls.

Motor Vehicle Crashes

The number of licensed drivers over age 65 is increasing. Currently, those over age 65 with driver's licenses represent about 13% of the drivers, and their crash rate is second only to the 16- to 25-year-old group. Persons over age 75 years have the highest rate of fatal crashes (Moore et al., 2004). Additionally many older adults are killed as pedestrians when struck by a motor vehicle.

Most MVCs involving older adults occur in the daytime, good weather, and close to home. Alcohol intoxication is much less frequent than in younger persons.

Contributing factors to automobile accidents by older adult patients are decreased coordination and reaction time, visual impairment, alterations in hearing processing, deficits in cognitive functioning, and antecedent medical conditions.

Burns

About 8% of the injury-related deaths to older persons are from burns. Burn injuries in older adults, compared to the younger population, are larger and deeper, and result in a greater mortality rate (Moore et al., 2004). Factors involved in older adult burns are altered mobility limiting muscle strength and coordination, which cause spilling and scalding; neurosensory changes, including peripheral neuropathy and vascular disease, causing alterations in sensation perception that allow prolonged contact with heat; forgetfulness and poor judgment regarding safety issues; and altered gait, limiting escape.

Decreased dermal cell production causes thinner skin, which allows burning to be more severe and susceptible to infection. Preexisting disease often make it impossible for the injured person to overcome serious but potentially survivable burns.

Elder Abuse

Abuse is a problem gaining more recognition, and older adult injuries must be carefully documented and investigated. Frequent visits for "minor" injuries, multiple bruises in various stages of coloration and healing, unkempt appearance, poor nutrition, and poor hygiene are all signals of possible abuse or neglect (see Table 14-1). Elder abuse is often not recognized and goes underreported.

TABLE 14-1: ELDER ABUSE ASSESSMENT

Unexplained dehydration

Unexplained poor nutrition

Unexplained bruises, wounds, or burns in various stages of healing

Unexplained fractures

Overmedication with sedatives

Disinterest exhibited by caregivers

Observed fear, withdrawal, or verbal confrontation between caregiver and patient

CHANGES CAUSED BY AGING

With aging, anatomic, physiologic, and mental changes occur. Resources diminish. Potential for healing diminishes (see Figure 14-1).

Cardiovascular System

Fibrosis causes progressive stiffening of the myocardium that results in diminished pump function and lower cardiac output. Blood pressure gradually increases. Blood vessels tend to harden.

Decreasing sensitivity to catecholamines, such as epinephrine and norepinephrine, causes an inability to develop appropriate tachycardia. Therefore, there is a decreased ability to increase cardiac output in response to hypovolemia, pain, and stress.

Older adult patients who have preexisting anemia and then sustain trauma may have a decrease in oxygen transport, which can precipitate angina or a myocardial infarction.

Respiratory System

Diminished pulmonary compliance and reduction of the ability to cough effectively are the result of decreased lung elasticity and progressive stiffening of the chest wall. Vital capacity of the lungs decreases.

FIGURE 14-1: CHANGES CAUSED BY AGING

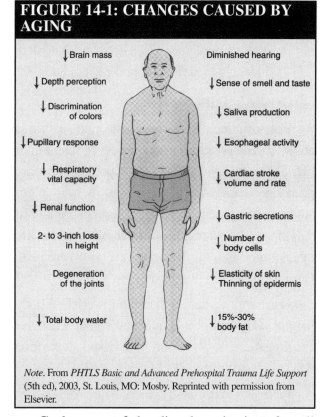

↓ Brain mass

↓ Depth perception

↓ Discrimination of colors

↓ Pupillary response

↓ Respiratory vital capacity

↓ Renal function

2- to 3-inch loss in height

Degeneration of the joints

↓ Total body water

Diminished hearing

↓ Sense of smell and taste

↓ Saliva production

↓ Esophageal activity

↓ Cardiac stroke volume and rate

↓ Gastric secretions

↓ Number of body cells

↓ Elasticity of skin Thinning of epidermis

↓ 15%-30% body fat

Note. From *PHTLS Basic and Advanced Prehospital Trauma Life Support* (5th ed), 2003, St. Louis, MO: Mosby. Reprinted with permission from Elsevier.

Coalescence of alveoli and a reduction of small airways support lead to a decrease in surface area for gas exchange. The reduced efficiency in gas exchange decreases arterial oxygenation.

Nervous System

Starting in the 40s, the brain begins to atrophy. By the 70s, there is a 10% reduction in the size of the brain. As a result, the space between the surface of the brain and the skull increases and stretches the dural bridging veins. The stretching of the veins makes them more vulnerable to disruption and bleeding commonly seen in subdural hematomas.

Functional deterioration of the following increases the potential for accidental injury:

*   Cognition
    — Poor memory, impaired judgment, and deficient data acquisition.
*   Hearing
    — Decreased auditory acuity, particularly with high-frequency sounds. Lack of or inadequate hearing devices due to financial limitations or limited access to health care.

- Eyesight
  — Decreased visual acuity and peripheral vision; intolerance to glare; and outdated, inadequate, or inappropriate eyeglasses.

Musculoskeletal System

Loss of bone density from osteoporosis brings about a predisposition to fractures, even with minor traumatic energy transfer. Osteoporosis is more pronounced in women but occurs in most older adults, leaving them prone to fractures especially of the hip and femur. Pelvic fractures can be life threatening and all fractures are slow to heal. Complications are not uncommon.

Osteoarthritis and diminution in vertebral body height contribute to significant spinal changes. Examples are kyphoscoliosis and spinal stenosis due to osteoarthritis.

Fibrosis and decrease in muscle mass diminishes agility and strength.

Renal System

Renal mass and function declines. By age 65, a 30-40% loss is not uncommon. Remaining nephrons show aging and deterioration on the tubules and glomeruli.

Sodium tends to be lost, and potassium tends to be retained. Potentially nephrotoxic agents, such as iodinated contrast solutions, aminoglycosides, and diuretics, should be used judiciously.

Metabolic and Hepatic Changes

The basal metabolic rate slows, along with the liver's ability to clear toxins. The caloric needs of men and women decline with age as lean body mass and metabolic rate gradually decrease. There is often chronic inadequate nutrition among older adults, which contributes to a significantly increased complication rate in geriatric trauma. Older adults also have a blunted immune response with resultant impaired ability to respond to infection and are more prone to develop multiple organ system failure.

Thermoregulation

The skin and connective tissues of older adults undergo extensive changes, including cell number decrease, loss of strength, and impaired function. Older adults therefore are more prone to heat loss, chilling, and dehydration than younger persons.

COMORBID CONDITIONS

Along with the anatomic and physiologic changes that occur in aging, significant diseases commonly develop and may seriously affect the older person's response to injury and stress.

It is essential for the nurse to find out concurrent diseases and medications in order for appropriate interventions and treatment to be administered. The information is important, and affects patient management, from resuscitation strategies to continuing care.

The more common conditions include cardiac disease, hypertension, neurologic disorders, liver disease, pulmonary disease, renal disease, diabetes, malignancy, and obesity.

COMMON INJURIES IN OLDER ADULTS

Hip and Femur Fractures

Osteoporosis contributes to the increase in long bone fractures seen in older adults. Long bone fractures in older adult patients are associated with prolonged disability and pulmonary morbidity and mortality. Early operative stabilization with aggressive management of the hemodynamic status have been shown to decrease morbidity and mortality.

Brain Injuries

Older adults have a higher incidence of subdural hematomas by three to one, compared to the younger population (American College of Surgeons, 2004b). This may be due to the higher use of anticoagulants in older adult patients and also to the physiology of aging on the brain. With atrophy of the brain there is a corresponding increased stretching of the parasagittal bridging veins, which make them more prone to rupture on impact causing the subdural hematoma. This can happen with even the most minor jarring of the body, like simply brushing up against a door frame while walking through the house. The patient and family often report that there was no history of trauma, which further confuses the clinical picture.

Burns

Burns are the third leading cause of traumatic death in older adults. Factors associated with degenerative disease and physical impairment appears to contribute significantly to the overrepresentation of burns in older adults. A small burn in an older adult with comorbid conditions may be a life-threatening event, while a large burn in a young person, is often survivable.

Rib Fractures

The mortality rate for chest injuries in older adult patients is higher than in non-older adult patients. Chest wall injury and rib fractures or pulmonary contusions are common and not well tolerated. Simple pneumothorax and hemothorax are of major concern and admission to the hospital is required. Pain control and vigorous pulmonary toilet are essential for a satisfactory outcome.

EVALUATION AND MANAGEMENT OF THE OLDER ADULT TRAUMA PATIENT

Primary Survey

As in all trauma cases, the ABCs are the initial approach for the older adult trauma patient. However, the following differences for the work-up of the older adult trauma patient should be emphasized.

- Supplemental oxygen should be administered to all older adult trauma patients even with the history of chronic obstructive pulmonary disease (COPD).
  - Continue to carefully monitor the patient because those with COPD retain carbon dioxide and lose the normal respiratory drive produced by an elevated $Paco_2$ level. Be prepared to intubate if necessary.

- Early aggressive intubation is warranted in older adult patients due to the limitation often seen in cardiopulmonary reserve. The presence of decreased level of consciousness and chest injury also warrants early aggressive intubation.

- Remove broken dentures but leave intact well-fitting dentures, as this will help achieve a good seal when using the valve bag mask.

- Use caution when inserting nasogastric tubes due to fragile tissues.

- All other principles of airway management remain the same.

- Early aggressive monitoring of the cardiovascular system is required.

- Expected vital sign changes that occur with shock may not be present because of medications that the patient is taking, such as a beta-blocker or calcium channel blocker.

- Evaluate blood pressure and heart rate in the context of the aged (see Table 14-2).

Pitfalls

- The older adult patient requires early and aggressive hemodynamic monitoring to identify those patients at risk for deterioration. Physiologic reserve is limited in older adult patients, making it difficult to generate an adequate response to injury.

- Central venous pressure monitoring, as well as pulmonary artery catheter insertion and monitoring, may be helpful along with traditional resuscitation endpoints, such as urine output and base deficit.

TABLE 14-2: PITFALLS IN THE INTERPRETATION OF VITAL SIGNS IN OLDER ADULT PATIENTS	
"Normal" Blood Pressure	A typical mistake with older adult patients is to believe that "normal" blood pressure and heart rate indicate normovolemia. Early and aggressive monitoring of the cardiovascular system is necessary. Blood pressure increases with age. Therefore, 120 mm Hg may represent hypotension in the older adult patient, whose normal pre-injury blood pressure was 170 mm Hg.
"Normal" Heart Rate	Absence of tachycardia. The older adult patient cannot generate an increased heart rate in response to blood loss. Therefore ongoing blood loss may be masked by the absence of tachycardia resulting in delayed diagnosis and poor outcome.

- Fluid resuscitation, while often necessary, should be done with care, especially with the cardiac patients. Lactated Ringer's solution is the initial fluid of choice.

- Careful monitoring of the electrolytes, blood sugar, blood urea nitrogen, and creatinine is warranted.

- Increased potential for medication toxicity is due to altered absorption of medications secondary to lean body mass and decreased liver and kidney function.

- Prolonged emergency department times are to be avoided. Shortened emergency department stays have been shown to improve the resuscitation of the older adult trauma patient.

- Avoiding unnecessary radiologic studies and moving the patient quickly to the intensive care unit for aggressive resuscitation, monitoring, and warming have proven beneficial to this special population.

- The optimal hemoglobin level for the older adult patient remains disputed. Age over 65 and the presence of cardiac disease are indications to maintain hemoglobin over 10 gm to maximize oxygen-carrying capacity. However, indiscriminate administration of blood is also to be avoided.

- If bleeding abdominal injury is suspected, early aggressive operation is warranted.

- Nonoperative management of spleen and liver injuries while aggressively pursued in all other age groups is not the standard of care in older adult patients. The older adult patient has little tolerance for blood loss and masks it to the degree that it can be dangerous to employ nonoperative management.

History

The initial assessment is a systematic search for serious injuries. The secondary assessment involves special attention to the history before the injury. This is crucial to appropriate management of the patient, possibly preventing inappropriate treatment or contributing to a potentially preventable event.

- Did an MVC occur under "normal" situations, or was there an antecedent episode, such as a cerebrovascular accident, a transient ischemic attack, or a myocardial infarction that caused the accident?

- Have more than one of these incidents or similar incidents occurred in the recent past? If so, there may be an untreated medical condition contributing to the incidents.

- Has the patient recently begun a new medication or had a change in the dosage of a regular medication?

- Get a list of all the patient's medications, dosages, and times of administration as soon as possible. If no one has a list, try to obtain all the patient's medication containers or call his pharmacy for a list (see Table 14-3).

Trauma in older adults requires a high level of expertise to generate good outcomes. Prompt transfer to a trauma center may be life saving.

END-OF-LIFE DECISIONS

Many older adult patients survive illnesses and injury and return to their previous level of function and independence. However, many struggle to rebound from the traumatic event. Long length of hospital stay with ventilator dependency and multiple complications are not infrequent in this population. There are times when the health care team in conjunction with the patient and family may choose to forgo life saving measures. This is particularly true in the case of extensive burns in advanced age, which has shown to be 100% nonsurvivable.

The trauma team should attempt to check for the existence of a living will, advance directives, or similar legal documents. Decisions should always be made in the best interest of the patient.

SUMMARY

Older persons are living longer and in better health than ever before. By the year 2020, the number of people in this country over age 65 will be at least 52 million.

The changes that occur with aging are anatomic, physiologic, and mental. These changes make identification of injury and recovery more complicated and long-term.

Trauma in older adults is likely to be more serious, develop more complications, be more costly and have more psychosocial ramifications than in the younger person. Early aggressive resuscitation and monitoring of the injured geriatric patient are necessary for improved outcomes.

TABLE 14-3: MEDICATIONS AND OLDER ADULT PATIENTS	
Drug	**Effect on Traumatic Injury**
Beta-Blockers	Limits the ability of the heart to generate a tachycardia which will mask shock
Calcium Channel Blockers	Prevents peripheral vasoconstriction and contributes to hypotension
Nonsteroidal Anti-inflammatory Agents	Affects platelet function, which contributes to blood loss
Chronic anticoagulants	Increases blood loss
Chronic diuretics	Dehydration contributing to shock

EXAM QUESTIONS

CHAPTER 14

Questions 86-94

86. Trauma in the older patient is likely to be

    a. less complicated than in younger persons.

    b. from abuse.

    c. the result of carelessness.

    d. more serious than the same injury seen in a younger person.

87. In the older person, the cardiovascular system changes include

    a. a progressive stiffening of the myocardium.

    b. decreased blood pressure.

    c. increased sensitivity to catecholamines.

    d. increased heart rate.

88. The most common mechanism of injury in persons over age 75 is

    a. motor vehicle crashes.

    b. falls.

    c. gunshot wounds.

    d. ingestion of a foreign body.

89. A patient presents with multiple bruises in various stages of healing. They are located on his upper arms. He also complains of neck pain. There are what appears to be round burn marks on his hands. His caregiver says he fell out of his wheelchair. The priority action for the nurse is to

    a. systematically assess the patient from head to toe for signs and symptoms of abuse.

    b. immediately report the caregiver to the authorities.

    c. evict the family from the hospital.

    d. have social services put a seat belt on the patient's wheelchair for his safety.

90. A head injury seen in the older adult patient is best characterized by

    a. epidural hematomas are the most common head injury seen.

    b. minor forms of trauma can result in significant head injury.

    c. brain atrophy contributes to susceptibility to infections.

    d. hormonal blood changes result in increased clotting.

91. The most common area for fracture in geriatric trauma is the

    a. hip.

    b. wrist.

    c. forearm.

    d. ankle.

92. In the older adult patient, shock can be masked by

    a. increased cerebral blood flow.

    b. lack of tachycardic response.

    c. peripheral vasodilation.

    d. increased lung vital capacity.

93. Which of the following should NOT be done during the initial assessment?

    a. Assess for unexplained dehydration or malnutrition.

    b. Assess the patient's pre-injury history.

    c. Ask the caregiver if they want to withhold treatment.

    d. Get a list of the patient's medications.

94. Beta-blockers

    a. may diminish the tachycardic response to trauma.

    b. cause peripheral vascular dilation.

    c. elevate blood pressure.

    d. constrict cranial blood vessels.

CHAPTER 15

PSYCHOSOCIAL CONSIDERATIONS

CHAPTER OBJECTIVE

Upon completion of this chapter, the reader will be able to identify the psychosocial issues affecting patients and families who have experienced a traumatic injury and also the staff taking care of trauma patients.

LEARNING OBJECTIVES

Upon completion of this chapter, the reader should be able to

1. describe three critical factors in crisis intervention on the trauma patient.

2. identify common psychosocial needs of the trauma patient.

3. recognize characteristics of posttraumatic stress disorder.

4. identify interventions for successful family presence during resuscitation.

5. specify interventions to optimize organ donation after trauma.

6. identify the principles of critical incident stress debriefing.

INTRODUCTION

A traumatic injury is a devastating event that produces both physical and psychological injury. Caring for the trauma patient includes having

a basic understanding of the psychosocial responses and needs the patient and significant others are likely to experience. The nurse, along with other members of the trauma team plays a significant role in assisting the patient and family to survive the crisis experience. Specific strategies can be used to support the patient and his family.

POTENTIAL FOR GROWTH OUT OF CRISIS

Trauma often occurs rapidly and is unanticipated. Both the patient and family are affected; often feeling vulnerable and ill prepared to deal with the event. As a result of the stress, coping mechanisms are called upon to adapt. If the coping mechanisms are inadequate there will be ongoing crisis. However, it is possible to not only recover to the previous level of functioning but also actually grow to a higher level of functioning. The crisis effectively managed can strengthen adaptive capacity, promote growth and learning, and enhance problem-solving abilities. Nurses can assist with appropriate interventions to achieve this higher growth (see Figure 15-1).

CRISIS INTERVENTION

Crisis intervention incorporates three important factors of crisis: 1) perception of the event, 2) adequacy of situational supports, and 3) effective-

FIGURE 15-1: POTENTIAL GROWTH CURVE OF CRISIS

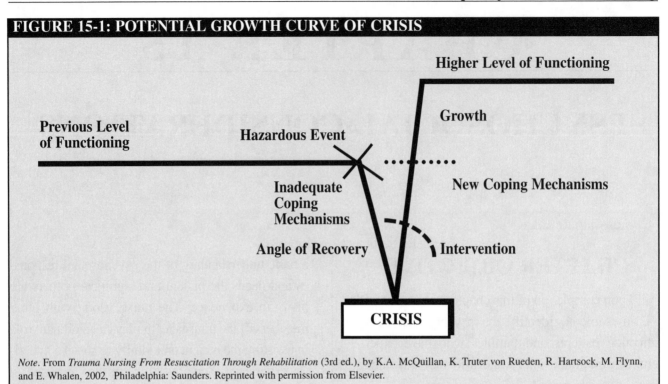

Note. From *Trauma Nursing From Resuscitation Through Rehabilitation* (3rd ed.), by K.A. McQuillan, K. Truter von Rueden, R. Hartsock, M. Flynn, and E. Whalen, 2002, Philadelphia: Saunders. Reprinted with permission from Elsevier.

ness of coping mechanisms (Aguilera, 1998). These factors often determine if an event will produce a crisis for individuals involved (see Table 15-1).

PSYCHOSOCIAL NEEDS

Several psychosocial needs have been identified as commonly occurring in patient and families suffering from trauma. These include the need for 1) information, 2) compassionate care, and 3) hope (see Table 15-2).

POSTTRAUMATIC STRESS DISORDER

Posttraumatic stress disorder (PTSD) is recognized as a major health concern after trauma. Historically, military phrases such as "battle fatigue" and "shell shocked" precede the now more common term posttraumatic stress disorder. Symptoms of PTSD can begin anytime after the event and persist for months. The following are typical signs and symptoms of PTSD:

TABLE 15-1: CRISIS INTERVENTION CRITICAL FACTORS

Factor	Nursing Intervention
Perception of the Event	• Clarify the individuals perception of the immediate event. • Ask "What does this mean to you." • Ask "Do you understand what was just explained."
Situational Supports	• Help the person identify people, agencies or things that have provided support in past situations. • Assist the person to establish contact with family, friends and or work associates for support.
Coping	• Help the patient to identify coping mechanisms used successfully in the past. Examples include: prayer, pets, music, exercise, discussion, or crying.

(Aguilera, 1998)

TABLE 15-2: PSYCHOSOCIAL NEEDS OF TRAUMA PATIENTS AND FAMILY	
Need	**Nursing Interventions**
Information	• Continually ask if they have questions. • Ask them to repeat what the physician has told them. • Provide clear, consistent, repeated explanations. • Ask them to repeat back to confirm understanding. • Encourage them to write down questions for the physician in advance of rounds. • Schedule regular patient/family/physician meetings.
Compassionate Care	• Use compassionate touch and tone of voice. • Refer to the patients by name. • Work to keep patient's pain under control. • Encourage the family to touch and talk to the patient. • Involve family in care as appropriate.
Hope	• No matter how critical the situation, allow the patient and family to hope.

- Intense fear, grief, anger, helplessness, or horror

- Sudden intense memories or flashback of the event

- Exhibit avoidance behavior or withdrawal from family and friends

- Appearance of being cold, indifferent, or pre-occupied

- Frequent biologic alarm reaction (for example, being jumpy around loud noises)

- Panic attacks when in situations that remind them of the traumatic event

- Frequent somatic complaints, such as gastric upset, headaches, irritability, difficulty concentrating, and insomnia.

All trauma patients experiencing a traumatic event, which they perceive to be stressful, should be screened for PTSD as soon as possible. Timing is critical because the faster the patient receives intervention the better the chance for recovery (McQuillan et al., 2002). Many trauma centers have psychological professionals assigned to the trauma unit, which are consulted acutely while the patient is still in the intensive care unit. Interventions for PTSD include pharmacologic measures and formal counseling sessions by trained psychiatric professionals with involvement of the family to ensure additional support.

FAMILY PRESENCE DURING RESUSCITATION

The frequency of family presence during resuscitation is on the rise. It is highly controversial and as yet is not embraced by most physician groups. Many professional nursing organizations however advocate for this change.

Research reveals that family members who were included in resuscitation attempts of sudden cardiac deaths viewed it as a positive experience. Families who witness resuscitation are reported to suffer fewer symptoms of grief and distress during the first 6 months of their bereavement. The idea of having family members in the resuscitation often stimulates trepidation in nurses and physicians. There is no evidence to suggest that lawsuits increase from this practice.

It should be noted that the majority of research has been conducted on cardiac patients and little is known if the same results would exist in trauma.

The reaction of families seeing their loved one disfigured with overt visual signs of trauma in addition to observing the resuscitation has yet to be studied. Individual hospitals have reported instituting this on a case-by-case basis, often being dependent on circumstances such as family members control and comfort level of the involved staff at the time (McQuillan et al., 2002).

Tips to Incorporate Family Presence During Resuscitation

- Offer the family the choice of being present. Avoid passing judgment and causing feelings of guilt, whatever their choice.

- Establish ground rules
  - The family will always be accompanied by a nurse.
  - The family can leave and return to the room at any time.
  - The family must not interfere with care for the good of the patient.
  - The family will be allowed to touch the patient as soon as it is practical.

- Assign a nurse specifically to the family during the resuscitation. This nurse should be experienced in handling distressed and grieving persons.

- Provide clear and honest explanations of all events.

- Tell the family when the patient is dead.

- Inform the family that they will be escorted from the room briefly while equipment is removed after which they can return to grieve in private.

- Provide the family the gift of time.
  - Allow the family time to reflect on the events.
  - Allow the family to ask further questions.

ORGAN DONATION

One of the country's most pressing public health concerns is the widening gap between the supply and demand for organs and tissues. Over 85,000 people in the nation are currently waiting for an organ. The United States is far from maximizing its supply of available organs from deceased donors. In 2003, organs were donated by only 6,455 of an estimated 14,000 potential donors (about 46%). *AS A RESULT, AN AVERAGE OF 17 PEOPLE ON THE TRANSPLANTATION WAITING LIST DIE EACH DAY* (U.S. Department of Health and Human Services, 2004).

General Facts About Organ Donation

- The donor's condition and care is always the first priority.

- There are no expenses to the donor's family related to transplantation. The recipient pays the costs.

- Recovery of tissues and organs is conducted under sterile surgical conditions, no different than any other surgical procedure.

- Once the tissues and organs are recovered, the ventilator is turned off, wounds are closed, and the body is released to the morgue, and then the funeral home.

- There is no disfigurement from the recovery process, so that an open casket funeral can be held.

- Identities of the donor and recipient are not disclosed. The donor's family will be told general information about the recipient, such as age, sex, and general geographic location.

A new initiative promoted by the Health and Human Services Department called the **Organ Donation Breakthrough Collaborative** (2004) intends to dramatically increase access to transplantable organs in the United States. Its purpose is to generate significant, measurable increases in organ donation by helping organ procurement organizations and large hospitals quickly identify, learn, adapt, replicate, and celebrate best practices that are associated with higher donation. A systems approach to organ donation is expected to be much more successful than the past approach of individuals attempting on their own to make an individual difference.

Drawing from the experience of practitioners with high donation rates, teams will work together to learn, adapt, redesign, test, and track their organ donation processes. The intent is to spread the information to the top 200 largest hospitals in the country. It is estimated that about 50% of the nations eligible donors are in the 200 largest hospitals. The goal is to achieve an average donation rate of 75% in these large hospitals, which will save or enhance thousands of more lives each year.

Suggested Strategies to Increase Organ Donation

1. Actively work to dispel myths surrounding organ donation with continued and repeated credible information.

2. Establish a "go to" person in your hospital who is knowledgeable about donation that staff can easily consult with when they are unsure about making a referral for organ donation.

3. Establish a strong relationship with the donor family early on and earn their trust.

4. Match same race requestors for families of same race and ethnicity when at all possible.

5. Conduct regular death record reviews to identify those with the highest donor potential and determine ways to increase donation.

To be successful, organ donation processes and protocols need to be implemented both within and outside of the hospital setting by champions from among organ procurement staff, hospital staff, and others such as medical examiners, EMS staff, and donor families. These processes and protocols span hospital development activities; family support and bereavement care, clinical support of potential donors, and follow-up.

CRITICAL INCIDENT STRESS DEBRIEFING

At times staff members have been involved with the treatment of trauma patients that causes them to react with unusually strong emotions. These critical incidents put staff at risk for continued dysfunction unless intervention is offered.

Critical incidents in trauma include:

- Death or homicide of a child

- Events that are associated with significant media presence

- Victims who are relatives or friends of a trauma team member

- Events that threaten the safety or lives of trauma team members

- Mass casualty situations

Critical incident stress management includes the use of debriefing techniques. These techniques include the gathering of staff after a stressful situation where emotions and information is shared. This allows for a safe, supportive environment where feelings can be expressed and performance analyzed without criticism. This promotes return to a productive level of functioning.

Critical Incident Stress Debriefing Measures

- Provide a debriefing as soon as possible (within 24 to 72 hours of the event)

- The session should be lead by trained personnel, usually mental health professionals and peer support personnel.

- Individuals are encouraged to discuss their role in the event and share how they felt during the incident and how they personalized the experience.

- Stress management strategies should be discussed and methods identified to support one another.

- Referrals are made as appropriate.

SUMMARY

Injury is physically and emotionally disrupting for the patient and family. Care of the injured patient includes psychosocial considerations. The psychological impact of the injury must be addressed throughout the trauma cycle. Timely application of crisis interventions assists the patient and the family as they deal with the stresses of the injury. The trauma nurse should take these considerations into account while providing trauma interventions. It is also important to include the family in support strategies. Often community agencies and other resources are necessary to support the patient from the point of injury through the rehabilitation process.

EXAM QUESTIONS

CHAPTER 15

Questions 95-100

95. Which of the following is a critical factor in crisis intervention? The patient's

    a. level of education.

    b. sex.

    c. age.

    d. support systems.

96. Mr. Jones is 80 years old and has just suffered a stroke. He is admitted to your intensive care unit and placed on a ventilator. Mr. Jones' son, Tom, arrives from out of state and is anxiously pacing outside of the waiting room. Which of the following statements regarding his psychosocial needs is true?

    a. The need for acceptance from the staff is paramount.

    b. The need to ventilate emotions is priority.

    c. The need for information while maintaining hope is important.

    d. The need to be with the patient is more important than the need for information.

97. In posttraumatic stress disorder

    a. the imprint of the traumatic moment can cause flashbacks.

    b. initial presenting symptoms often do not occur until years after the event.

    c. treatment is more effective if held until the patient moves to rehabilitation.

    d. the patient often draws closer to his family and friends as a means to cope.

98. A 34-year-old male motorcyclist who was hit by a car arrives to the trauma center in full arrest. Initial assessment reveals blown pupils, blood per mouth, nose and ears with a GCS of 3. There are no other signs of trauma to the body. The patient is intubated and IVs started. The patient deteriorates into ventricular fibrillation and is unable to be shocked out of the rhythm and expires on the table. The wife is hovering in the hallway outside of the resuscitation room. Which of the following would have the greatest impact on meeting the wife's needs?

    a. Call pastoral care or a social worker to come and provide counseling.

    b. Tell the wife that her husband has expired and that she can see him as soon as the staff cleans up the room and removes the equipment.

    c. Suggest that she may not want to view the patient due to obvious injuries.

    d. Assign a nurse to meet the wife, explain the situation, and offer the opportunity to see the patient.

99. Successful strategies to increase organ donation include

    a. public educational seminars.

    b. education of the nursing staff to support families in crisis.

    c. increased availability of financial information regarding donation.

    d. establishing a local hospital expert "go to person" on donation.

100. Critical incident debriefing might be required for

    a. Joint Commission on Accreditation of Healthcare Organizations approval.

    b. death of a 7-year-old child shot by a fellow classmate at school.

    c. death of a 60-year-old cancer patient.

    d. all emergency department deaths.

This concludes the final examination.

RESOURCES

Ahrns, K. (2004). Trends in burn resuscitation: shifting the focus from fluids to adequate endpoint monitoring, edema control, and adjuvant therapies. *Critical Care Nursing Clinics North America, 16*(1), 75-98.

American Trauma Society (2005). The Trauma Information Exchange Program (TIEP). www.amtrauma.org/tiep

Arbour, R. (2004). Intracranial hypertension: monitoring and nursing assessment. *Critical Care Nurse, 24*(5), 19-34.

Barry, M. (2001). Ankle sprains. *American Journal Nursing, 101*(10), 40-42.

Bernardo, L. (2002). Emergency nurses role in pediatric injury prevention. *Nursing Clinics of North America, 37*(1), 135-143.

Brettler, S. (2004). Traumatic brain injury. *Registered Nurse, 67*(4), 32-38.

Bushard, S. (2002). Trauma in patients who are morbidly obese. *Association periOperative Registered Nurses, 76*(4), 585-589.

Campbell, P., Dennie, M., Dougherty, K., Iwaskiw, O., & Rollo, K. (2004). Implementation of an ED protocol for pain management at triage at a busy level I trauma center. *Journal Emergency Nurses, 30*(5), 431-438.

Cassabaum, V. (2002). The ins and outs of renal trauma. *American Journal Nursing,* September (Suppl.), 34-36.

Chavis, S. & Duncan, L. (2003). Pain management continuum of care for surgical patients. *Association periOperative Registered Nurses, 78*(3), 381-404.

Clontz, A., Annonio, D., & Walker, L. (2004). Amputation, *Registered Nurse, 67*(7), 38-44.

Danks, R. & Danks, B. (2003). Laryngeal mask airway: review of indications and use. *Journal Emergency Nursing, 30*(1), 30-35.

DeBaer, S. & O'Connor, A. (2004). Prehospital and emergency department burn care. *Critical Care Nursing Clinics of North America, 16*(1), 61-73.

Fitzpatrick, M. (2002). A new tool for initial stabilization of pelvic fractures: the TPOD trauma pelvic orthotic device. *Journal of Trauma Nursing, 9*(1), 20-22.

Frakes, M. (2003). Rapid sequence induction medications: an update. *Journal Emergency Nursing, 29*(6), 533-539.

Frakes, M. & Evans, T. (2004). Major pelvic fractures. *Critical Care Nurse, 24*(2), 18-32.

Hilton, G. (2001). Acute head injury. *American Journal Nursing, 101*(9), 51-52.

Hilton, G. (2001). Thermal burns. *American Journal Nursing, 101*(11), 32-34.

Holleran, R. (2002). The problem of pain in emergency care. *Nursing Clinics of North America, 37*(1), 67-78.

Hubble, M. & Hubble, J. (2002). *Principles of Advanced Trauma Care.* Albany, NY: Delmar Thomson Learning.

Ihlenfeld, J. (2003). A primer on triage and mass casualty events. *Dimensions Critical Care Nurse, 22*(5), 204-209.

Infante, M. (1982). *Crisis theory: a framework for nursing practice.* Englewood Cliffs, NJ: Prentice Hall.

Ingram, J. & Rayburn, A. (2002). Critical care nurses' attitudes and knowledge related to organ donation. *Dimensions Critical Care Nurse, 21*(6), 249-255.

Jagim, M. (2003). Emergency airway management. *American Journal Nursing, 103*(10), 32-35.

Kleinpell, R. (2003). The role of the critical care nurse in assessment and management of the patient with severe sepsis. *Critical Care Clinics North America, 15*(1), 27-34.

Koestner, A. (2001). Spinal cord injury without radiographic abnormality (SCIWORA) in children. *Journal of Trauma Nursing, 8*(4), 101-108.

LaBorde, P. (2004). Burn epidemiology: the patient, the nation, the statistics, and the data resources. *Critical Care Nursing Clinics North America, 16*(1), 13-26.

Lafleur, K. (2004). Taking the 5th vital sign. *Registered Nurse, 67*(7), 30-37.

LeJeune, G. & Howard-Fain, T. (2002). Nursing assessment and management of patients with head injuries. *Dimensions Critical Care Nurse, 21*(6), 226-231.

Mayer, D.M., Torma, L., Byock, I., & Norris, K. (2001). Speaking the language of pain. *American Journal Nursing, 101*(2), 45-50.

McMahon, M. (2003). ED triage. *American Journal Nursing, 103*(3), 61-63.

Merrel, P. & Mayo, D. (2004). Inhalation injury in the burn patient. *Critical Care Nursing Clinics North America, 16*(1), 27-38.

Mikhail, J. (2004). Massive transfusion in trauma: process and outcomes. *Journal of Trauma Nursing, 11*(2), 55-60.

Mikhail, J. (1999a). Resuscitation endpoints in trauma. *American Association Critical Care Nurses Clinical Issues, 10*(1), 10-20.

Mikhail, J. (1999b). The triad of death: hypothermia, acidosis, and coagulopathy. *American Association Critical Care Nurses Clinical Issues, 10*(1), 85-93.

Milner, S. & Mottar, R. (2001). The burn wheel: an innovative method for calculating the need for fluid resuscitation in burned patients. *American Journal Nursing, 101*(11), 35-44.

Miracle, V. (2003). What every nurse should know about pain management. *Dimensions Critical Care Nursing, 22*(3), 133-134.

Montgomery, R. (2004). Pain management in burn injury. *Critical Care Nursing Clinics North America, 16*(1), 39-49.

Odhner, M., Wegman, D., Freeland, N., Steinmetc, A., & Ingersoll, G. (2003). Assessing pain control in nonverbal critically ill adults. *Dimensions Critical Care Nurses, 22*(6), 260-267.

Proehl, J. (2004). Accidental amputation. *American Journal Nursing, 104*(2), 50-53.

Ruffolo, D. (2002). Delayed splenic rupture understanding the threat. *Journal of Trauma Nursing, 9*(2), 34-40.

Rzucidlo, S. & Shirk, B. (2004). Trauma nursing of pediatric patients. *Registered Nurses, 67*(6), 36-42.

Scaletta, T. & Schaider, J. (2001). *Emergent Management of Trauma.* (2nd ed.) New York: McGraw Hill.

Schulman, C. (2002). End points of resuscitation: choosing the right parameters to monitor. *Dimensions Critical Care Nurse, 21*(1), 2-14.

Sicoutris, C. (2001). Management of hypothermia in the trauma patient. *Journal of Trauma Nursing, 8*(1), 5-15.

Smith, M. (2004). Unique considerations in caring for a pediatric burn patient: a developmental approach. *Critical Care Nursing Clinics North America, 16*(1), 99-108.

Thomas, D.O. (2002). Special considerations for pediatric triage in the emergency department. *Nursing Clinics of North America, 37*(1), 145-159.

Tucker, T.L. (2002). Family presence during resuscitation. *Critical Care Nursing Clinics North America, 14*, 177-185.

Urquhart, B. (2001). Anterior shoulder dislocation. *American Journal Nursing, 101*(2), 33-35.

Wagner, J. (2004). Lived experience of critically ill patients' family members during cardiopulmonary resuscitation. *American Journal of Critical Care, 13*(5), 416-420.

Williams, J. (2002). Family presence during resuscitation. *Nursing Clinics of North America, 37*(1), 211-220.

Wise, B., Mudd, S., & Wilson, M. (2002). Management of blunt abdominal trauma in children. *Journal Trauma Nursing, 9*(1), 6-14.

Wong, D. (2003). Pain control: topical local anesthetics. *American Journal Nursing, 103*(6) 42-46.

TRAUMA-RELATED WEB SITES

American Burn Association
www.ameriburn.org

American College of Surgeons
www.facs.org

American Trauma Society
www.amtrauma.org

Association for the Advancement of Automotive Medicine
www.carcrash.org

Glasgow Coma Score
www.trauma.org/scores/gcs.html

Gray's Anatomy Online
www.bartleby.com/107

Journal of Trauma
www.jtrauma.com

National Center for Injury Prevention and Control
www.cdc.gov/ncipc/default.htm

National Highway Traffic Safety Administration (NHTSA)
www.nhtsa.dot.gov

Organ Injury Scaling
www.trauma.org/scores/ois.html

Revised Trauma Scoring7
www.trauma.org/scores/rts.html

Society of Trauma Nurses
www.traumanursesoc.org

Trauma
www.trauma.org

GLOSSARY

acceleration injury: Any injury resulting from an acceleration or increased speed of the body forward.

Battle's sign: Ecchymosis over the mastoid area that may indicate a fracture at the base of the skull.

blunt trauma: Damage to the body without penetration of the skin, caused by rapid deceleration and sudden impact with an object.

brain death: Cessation of all functions of the entire brain, including the brain stem. Cerebral functions are absent. Brain stem functions are absent. The heart is kept beating by mechanical support, but the patient is not alive or being kept alive by the machines. The patient is not actually functioning or living.

burn: Tissue injury resulting from excessive exposure to thermal, chemical, electrical, or light mechanisms; smoke inhalation; or radiation. Effects vary according to the type of burn, duration of exposure, intensity of the agent, and the part of the body involved.

Beck's triad: Classic symptoms of cardiac tamponade which include distended neck veins, hypotension, and muffled heart tones.

cardiopulmonary resuscitation (CPR): An emergency technique used in the attempt to save the patient's life when he is in cardiac or respiratory arrest. The goal is to provide oxygen quickly to the brain, heart, and other vital organs until definitive medical treatment is able to restore cardiac and pulmonary functions.

cardiovascular system: A system comprised of the heart and blood vessels, including the aorta, arteries, arterioles, capillaries, venules, veins, and vena cava. The system keeps the body running by delivering oxygen and nutrients and disposing of cellular waste and carbon dioxide through a complex arrangement of systemic circulation and pulmonary circulation.

central nervous system (CNS): The portion of the nervous system made up of the brain and spinal cord. The brain is the controlling organ of the body and the spinal cord transmits messages back and forth between the brain and the body.

child maltreatment: Although different states' definitions vary to an extent, the terms child abuse and maltreatment are used interchangeably to describe neglect and/or physical, emotional, and/or sexual abuse to the child.

choroid: The dark-brown vascular coat of the eye between the sclera and retina. The choroid is made up of blood vessels united by connective tissue containing pigmented cells and five layers. It is a part of the uvea or vascular tunic of the eye.

comorbid conditions in elderly people: Diseases that commonly develop, along with the anatomic and physiologic changes occurring in aging, that seriously affect the elder person's response to injury.

compartment syndrome: increased pressure in a fascial compartment because of either an internal source, such as hemorrhage or edema, or an external source, such as a cast; nerves, blood vessels, and/or muscle can be compressed as pressure rises inside the compartment.

contrecoup injury: Injury occurring on the opposite side from the impact to the head.

coup injury: Injury on the same side of the impact to the head.

cranial nerves: Twelve pairs of nerves originating in the brain stem, each having a separate name, Roman numeral identifier, and anatomical and physiological function. The nerves have unconscious control over sensory, motor, or both activities.

Cushings triad: Increased systolic blood pressure, widened pulse pressure, and a reflex bradycardia as a response to cerebral and brain stem ischemia.

death: Irreversible cessation of circulatory and respiratory function, evidenced by persistent cessation of these functions. Time and date must be documented on the patient's medical record and signed by the physician.

deceleration injury: An injury resulting from a force that stops or decreases the velocity of a moving victim.

decerebrate posturing: Extension and internal rotation of the upper extremities, wrist flexion, and extension, internal rotation and plantar flexion of the lower extremities; usually bilateral; may represent significant injury to the midbrain and or pons.

decorticate posturing: Adduction of the shoulders, pronation and flexion of the elbows and wrists along with extremities; bilateral: may represent significant injury to the cerebrum or corticospinal motor tracts.

diffuse head injury: A head injury that involves the entire brain.

displaced fracture: A fractured bone that has been pushed out of alignment, causing deformity and requiring reduction before immobilization.

dyskinesia: Difficulty or distortion in performing voluntary movements.

embryo: The stage in prenatal development between being the ovum and becoming the fetus, lasting from the 2nd to 8th week of gestation.

epidemiology: The distribution and determinants of disease frequency in man. Epidemiology is relative to trauma in the collection of data such as age, gender, race/ethnicity, and geographic characteristics that form frequency and distribution patterns of injury, morbidity, and mortality due to trauma.

exsanguination: Extensive loss of blood due to internal or external hemorrhage.

failure to thrive: A condition seen in children under age 5 when growth continues to significantly fail to meet the norms for age and sex based on national growth charts.

flail chest: Abnormal chest wall movement, flail chest is two or more consecutive ribs broken in two or more places resulting in a portion of the rib cage becoming unstable and moving in a direction opposite the rest of the rib cage during inspiration and expiration.

fetus: The developing child in utero from the 3rd month of pregnancy to birth.

focal head injury: A head injury having a specific area of involvement.

foot pound: Work expended when 1 lb is moved a distance of 1 foot in the direction of the force.

gestation: The period of time from conception to birth, usually from 38-40 weeks.

Glasgow Coma Scale Score: A scoring system to measure the patient's level of consciousness; score ranges from 3 to 15; points correspond to responses in three areas: eye opening, verbal response, and motor response. The patient's best responses in each of three areas are added for a total score.

golden hour: Refers to the occurrence of death following injury as a function of time. There are three peaks of the occurrence of death after injury: immediate, early, and late. It is "early" deaths, occurring within the first few hours, that the "golden hour" refers to. Modern trauma centers are often able to save these patients. Survival of seriously injured or ill patients is the highest when intervention takes place within the first "golden hour" after the injury occurs.

inhalation injury: Damage to the air passages caused by the inhalation of toxic fumes, hot air, or carbon monoxide.

Kehr's sign: Referred left shoulder pain associated with splenic rupture because of blood irritating the phrenic nerve.

kinematics: Branch of mechanics that deals with the study of motion.

Level I trauma center: A hospital providing the highest level of trauma care and services 24 hours a day, 7 days a week. Injury prevention initiatives and trauma research required.

Level II trauma center: Hospital capabilities similar to Level I centers. The trauma team is not necessarily in-house 24 hours a day, but must be able to meet the severely injured patients when they arrive in the emergency department.

Level III trauma center: Hospitals that are not immediately accessible to Level I and II centers. In-house surgical coverage on a 24-hour basis is not required and staffing may be on an on-call basis. Accessibility to higher-level facilities should be timely and is often by helicopter transportation.

malocclusion: A misaligned bite caused by facial trauma to the jaw.

manual techniques to clear the airway: Techniques used to open the patient's airway, which include jaw thrust, head tilt-chin lift, and chin-lift maneuvers.

mechanical methods for airway control: Used in the semiconscious or unconscious patient when basic manual techniques do not clear the airway. Use of these mechanisms requires special training for professionals. Devices include oropharyngeal airways, nasopharyngeal airways, esophageal obturator airways, pharyngotracheal lumen airways, and endotracheal tubes.

meninges: Three vascular layers of membranes that surround and protect the brain and spinal cord.

Monro-Kellie hypothesis: A slight increase in any one of three volumes of the cranial cavity (brain, blood, cerebrospinal fluid) causes a decrease in another volume without a significant change in intracranial pressure.

neglect: Intentional or unintentional omission of needed care and support, or the caregiver being either unable or unwilling to provide the most basic needs for the person in his care.

nursing diagnosis: A clinical nursing judgment about individual, family, or community reactions or responses to illness or injury, problems, or life processes. The diagnoses serve as a basis for nursing interventions that have outcomes for which the nurse is accountable. The physician does not have to give an order for these interventions.

orbital complex: A bony pyramid-shaped cavity in the skull that contains and protects the eyes, comprised of the frontal bone, zygoma, and maxilla.

organ donor: After death has been pronounced, it is determined by the organ procurement agency, according to specified criteria, as to the patient's suitability for the donation of organs (and/or tissues) to be used in transplantation.

orthopedic injuries: Musculoskeletal injuries, including soft-tissue strains and sprains; damage to the skin, tendons, ligaments, cartilage, and associated vessels and nerves; and dislocations, subluxations, and fractures that are a significant cause of short- and long-term disabilities.

pathologic fracture: A fracture in a diseased or weak bone that can occur with minimal force. Pathologic fractures frequently occur in the spine without the patient being aware of the fracture; he "just gets shorter."

penetrating trauma: Injury caused by an object hitting the body with such force that it pierces the skin, and, which may leave tissue and organ injury or destruction along its path.

peripheral nervous system: Linking cables of nerve fibers reaching outside the central nervous system. The system includes the nerves that enter and leave the spinal cord and those that connect the brain and organs without passing through the spinal cord. There are 31 pairs of peripheral nerves called spinal nerves and 12 pairs of cranial nerves.

peritoneal space: A cavity that is really a potential space between the layers of the parietal and visceral peritoneum. It contains a small amount of fluid so that the viscera can glide easily on each other or against the wall of the abdominal cavity.

physical abuse: Intentional infliction of physical injury, torture, maiming, or unreasonable force, or omission/failure to protect the individual from danger and injury.

prehospital care: The part of the emergency medical services system beginning at the point of discovery of a person's illness or injury, access to the system, and professional medical care until the patient reaches the emergency department. There are two levels of care provided by prehospital personnel: basic life support (BLS) and advanced life support (ALS).

priapism: Abnormal, painful, and continued erection of the penis due to disease or may be due to lesions of the cord above the lumbar region.

primary assessment: Rapid and accurate initial assessment of the patient's condition that is conducted on every patient. Primary assessment includes determination of the status of the ABCs: airway, breathing, and circulation. Included are: Providing resuscitation and stabilization on a priority basis; determination of critical injuries, and the level of care the patient needs.

psychosocial: The internal/psychological and interpersonal/social factors that determine a person's emotional state. Psychosocial conditions should not be confused with psychiatric or altered mental conditions.

pulse pressure: The difference between the systolic and diastolic blood pressures. It roughly reflects the degree of vasoconstriction or vasodilation of the blood vessels.

raccoon's eyes: Black eyes or discoloration under the eyes that may indicate a basilar skull fracture.

respiratory system: A system consisting of air passages and organs: nasal cavities, oral cavity, pharynx, larynx, trachea, and lungs, including bronchi, bronchioles, alveolar ducts, and alveoli. The system functions to bring in and distribute oxygen to nourish the body and to rid it of the waste products of respiration.

response to trauma: Response to trauma going beyond the physical injury and including the mind and spirit's reactions; a complex, integrated system of reactions.

retinal detachment: The pigment layer of the retina, remains attached to the choroid and the rest of the retina detaches from it. Occurs with or without a tear.

retroperitoneal: Located behind the peritoneum and outside the peritoneal cavity, containing the kidneys, bladder, ureters, reproductive organs, inferior vena cava, and abdominal aorta.

saddle nose: A nose with a depressed bridge—usually congenital—due to the absence of bone or cartilidge support; due to disease; or it may be a deformity secondary to trauma causing a septal hematoma.

secondary assessment: Conducted after the primary assessment, or survey, is completed and the ABCs are stabilized. The purpose is to thoroughly evaluate and document additional injuries and illnesses, including stopping any bleeding and administering supplemental oxygen. The patient is reassessed frequently, and a history is obtained, along with recording the patient's current medications and allergies.

shock: A clinical syndrome that is a series of reactions to mental or physical upset of the body's internal balance.

thermoregulation: The regulation of temperature, and physiologically, body temperature.

trauma: Physical injury caused by an external action, such as an assaulting force, thermal, or chemical agent that is strong enough to potentially threaten a patient's limbs or life.

trauma center: A hospital facility designated according to the level of trauma care it provides. Determination is made according to established criteria regarding the numbers and qualifications of the surgeons who staff on a 24-hour-a-day basis and specialty services provided. Levels of trauma centers are I, II, and III. Trauma centers have a team activation system that operates according to triage criteria with its members having defined roles and responsibilities to provide systematic and coordinated care.

triage: Injury assessment using defined criteria. Triage means sorting. In emergency medical services, it means assessment to sort the patients by severity of illness or injury. The process is used in a prehospital situation where the patient is assessed and directed to the most appropriate level of hospital emergency services. In the emergency department, triage is used to sort the severity of illness or injury in order to determine the priority of care the patient receives. Triage is also used during mass casualties and military operations.

UNOS: United Network for Organ Sharing (UNOS) is a private, nonprofit agency that operates the Organ Procurement and Transplantation Network by serving as a clearinghouse and carrying out the objectives of the Secretary of the Department of Health and Human Services in accordance with the National Organ Transplantation Act of 1984.

urinary system: Controls the elimination of specific toxic waste products filtered from the blood, along with managing the body's water and electrolyte balance. Other functions include the stimulation of red blood cell production, activation of vitamin D, and insulin degradation.

BIBLIOGRAPHY

American College of Surgeons. (1997). *Advanced trauma life support® for doctors (ACLS®) student manual* (6th ed.). Chicago, IL: ACS.

American College of Surgeons. (2004a). *Advanced trauma life support® for doctors student course manual* (7th ed.). Chicago, IL: ACS.

American College of Surgeons. (2004b). *National trauma data bank annual report.* Retrieved August 11, 2005, from http://www.facs.org/trauma/ntdbannualreport2004.pdf

American College of Surgeons. (2004c). *National Trauma Databank Pediatric Report.* Retrieved October 28, 2005 from http://www.facs.org/trauma/ntdbpediatric2004.pdf

Aguilera, D. (1998). *Crisis intervention: theory and methodology* (8th ed.). St. Louis, MO: Mosby.

Bureau of Health Services Resources, Division of Trauma and Emergency Medical Services. (2000). Model trauma care system plan. *Health Resources and Services Administration,* U.S. Department of Health and Human Services, Rockville, MD.

Campbell, J. (Ed.) (2004). *Basic Trauma Life Support for advanced providers.* Upper Saddle River, NJ: Prentice Hall.

Davis, J., Parks, S., Kaups, K., Gladen, H., & O'Donnel-Nicol, S. (1996). Admission base deficit predicts transfusion requirements and risk of complications. *Journal of Trauma, 41,* 469-774.

DeDoer, A., Mintjes-deGroot, A., & Severignem, A. (1999). Risk assessment for surgical site infections in orthopedic patients. *Infection Control Hospital Epidemiology, 20*(6), 402-409.

Department of Health and Human Services, Health Resources and Services Administration. (1992). *Model Trauma Care System Plan.* Rockville, MD.

Donovan, A. (1994). *Trauma surgery techniques in thoracic, abdominal, and vascular surgery.* St. Louis, MO: Mosby-Year Book.

Ferrera, P., Colucciello, S., Marx, J., & Verdile, V., Gibbs, M. (2001). *Trauma management an emergency medicine approach.* St. Louis: Mosby.

Limmer, D., Elling, B., & O'Keefe, M. (2002). *Essentials of Emergency Care.* Upper Saddle River, NJ: Prentice Hall.

Limmer, D., O'Keefe, M.F., Grant, H.D., Murray, R.H., & Bergson, J.D. (2001). *Emergency Care.* Upper Saddle River, NJ: Brady Prentice Hall.

MacKenzie, E. (2003). National inventory of hospital trauma centers. *Journal American Medical Association, 289*(12), 1516-1519.

Mandavia, D.P., Newton, E.J., & Demetriades, D. (2003). *Color atlas of emergency trauma.* New York: Cambridge University Press.

McQuillan, K.A., Truter von Rueden, K., Hartsock, R., Flynn, M., & Whalen, E. (2002). *Trauma nursing from resuscitation through rehabilitation* (3rd ed.). Philadelphia: Saunders.

McSwain, N. & Frame, S. (Eds.) (2003). *Prehospital trauma life support.* National Association of Emergency Medical Technicians. St. Louis, MO: Mosby.

Mikhail, J. (2002). Backboard removal: guideline for trauma care. *Journal of Trauma Nursing, 9*(3), 73-74.

Moore, E., Feliciano, D., & Mattox, K. (2004). *Trauma* (5th ed.). New York: McGraw-Hill.

National Highway Traffic Safety Administration. (2000). National Standard Curriculum for Bystander Care. Retrieved August 20, 2005, from http://www.nhtsa.dot.gov/people /injury /ems /FirstThere

National Highway Traffic Safety Administration. (2002). Child Passenger Safety 2002. Retrieved August 20, 2004, from http://www.nhtsa.dot.gov/ CPS/ChildRestraints.html

O'Keefe, M., Limmer, D., Grant, H., Murray, R., & Bergerson, J. (2004). *Brady emergency care* (10th ed). Upper Saddle River, NJ: Brady Prentice Hall.

Peitzman, A., Rhodes, M., Schwab, C., Yealy, D., & Fabian, T. (2002). *The Trauma Manual* (2nd ed.). Philadelphia: Lippincott Williams & Wilkins.

Scaletta, T.A. & Schaider, J.J. (2001). *Emergent Management of Trauma* (2nd ed.). New York: McGraw-Hill.

U.S. Department of Health and Human Services. (2004). Organ donation breakthrough collaborative. Retrieved November 29, 2004, from http://organdonation.iqsolutions.com/

US Department of Transportation, National Highway Traffic Safety Administration (2005). Traffic Safety Facts 2004 Early Edition, Washington, DC. Retrieved December 8, 2005 from http://www-nrd.nhtsa.dot.gov/pdf/nrd-30/NCSA/TSFAnn/TSF2004EE.pdf#search='tr affic%20safety%20facts%202004'

Wills, M., Goold, G., & Watson, K. (2000). *Med EMT a learning system for prehospital care.* Upper Saddle River, NJ: Prentice Hall.

INDEX

PRETEST KEY

Principles of
Basic Trauma Nursing
2nd Edition

1.	a	Introduction & Chapter 1
2.	c	Chapter 1
3.	b	Chapter 2
4.	a	Chapter 3
5.	b	Chapter 3
6.	b	Chapter 4
7.	c	Chapter 4
8.	d	Chapter 5
9.	a	Chapter 5
10.	b	Chapter 6
11.	d	Chapter 6
12.	c	Chapter 7
13.	c	Chapter 7
14.	b	Chapter 8
15.	a	Chapter 8
16.	d	Chapter 9
17.	c	Chapter 9
18.	c	Chapter 10
19.	b	Chapter 11
20.	a	Chapter 12
21.	c	Chapter 13
22.	d	Chapter 13
23.	b	Chapter 14
24.	d	Chapter 15
25.	a	Chapter 15

Western Schools® offers over 1,900 hours to suit all your interests – and requirements!

Cardiovascular
Cardiovascular Nursing: A Comprehensive Overview ....32 hrs
A The 12-Lead ECG in Acute Coronary Syndromes ....42 hrs

Clinical Conditions/Nursing Practice
A Advanced Assessment ....35 hrs
Airway Management with a Tracheal Tube ....1 hr
Asthma: Nursing Care Across the Lifespan ....28 hrs
Auscultation Skills ....38 hrs
    — Heart Sounds...20 hrs
    — Breath Sounds...18 hrs
Chest Tube Management ....2 hrs
Clinical Care of the Diabetic Foot ....8 hrs
A Complete Nurses Guide to Diabetes Care ....37 hrs
Diabetes Essentials for Nurses ....30 hrs
Death, Dying & Bereavement ....30 hrs
Essentials of Patient Education ....30 hrs
Healing Nutrition ....24 hrs
Holistic & Complementary Therapies ....18 hrs
Home Health Nursing...30 hrs
Humor in Healthcare: The Laughter Prescription ....20 hrs
Orthopedic Nursing: Caring for Patients with
    Musculoskeletal Disorders ....30 hrs
Osteomyelitis ....2 hrs
Pain & Symptom Management ....1 hr
Pain Management: Principles and Practice ....30 hrs
A Palliative Practices: An Interdisciplinary Approach ....66 hrs
    — Issues Specific to Palliative Care ....20 hrs
    — Specific Disease States and Symptom
        Management ....24 hrs
    — The Dying Process, Grief, and
        Bereavement...22 hrs
Pharmacologic Management of Asthma ....1 hr
Seizures: A Basic Overview...1 hr
The Neurological Exam..1 hr
Wound Management and Healing ....30 hrs

Critical Care/ER/OR
Basic Nursing of Head, Chest, Abdominal, Spine
    and Orthopedic Trauma..20 hrs
A Case Studies in Critical Care Nursing ....46 hrs
Critical Care & Emergency Nursing ....30 hrs
Hemodynamic Monitoring ....18 hrs
A Nurse Anesthesia ....58 hrs
    — Common Diseases ....20 hrs
    — Common Procedures.....................................21 hrs
    — Drugs...17 hrs
A Practical Guide to Moderate Sedation/Analgesia.............31 hrs
Principles of Basic Trauma Nursing..................................30 hrs

Geriatrics
Alzheimer's Disease: A Complete Guide for Nurses ....25 hrs
Nursing Care of the Older Adult ....30 hrs
Psychosocial Issues Affecting Older Adults.....................16 hrs

Infectious Diseases/Bioterrorism
Avian Influenza ....1 hr
Biological Weapons ....5 hrs
Bioterrorism & the Nurse's Response to WMD..................5 hrs
Bioterrorism Readiness: The Nurse's Critical Role .... 2 hrs
Hepatitis C: The Silent Killer (2nd ed.) ....3 hrs
HIV/AIDS ....1 or 2 hrs
Infection Control Training for Healthcare Workers ....4 hrs
Influenza: A Vaccine-Preventable Disease..........................1 hr
MRSA ....1 hr
Smallpox..2 hrs
West Nile Virus (2nd ed.)...1 hr

Oncology
Cancer in Women ....30 hrs
Cancer Nursing (2nd ed.) ....36 hrs
Chemotherapy and Biotherapies ....10 hrs

Pediatrics/Maternal-Child/Women's Health
A Assessment and Care of the Well Newborn ....34 hrs
Attention Deficit Hyperactivity Disorders
    Throughout the Lifespan ....30 hrs
Diabetes in Children ....30 hrs
End-of-Life Care for Children and Their Families.............2 hrs
Induction of Labor ....8 hrs
Manual of School Health ....30 hrs
Maternal-Newborn Nursing ....30 hrs
Menopause: Nursing Care for Women
    Throughout Mid-Life ....25 hrs
A Obstetric and Gynecologic Emergencies ....44 hrs
    — Obstetric Emergencies ....22 hrs
    — Gynecologic Emergencies ....22 hrs
Pediatric Nursing: Routine to Emergent Care ....30 hrs
Pediatric Pharmacology ....10 hrs
Pediatric Physical Assessment ....10 hrs
A Practice Guidelines for Pediatric Nurse Practitioners ....46 hrs
Women's Health: Contemporary Advances and Trends ......30 hrs

Professional Issues/Management/Law
Documentation for Nurses ....24 hrs
Medical Error Prevention: Patient Safety ....2 hrs
Management and Leadership in Nursing ....20 hrs
Ohio Law: Standards of Safe Nursing Practice (3rd ed.) ....1 hr
Surviving and Thriving in Nursing...................................30 hrs
Understanding Managed Care ....30 hrs

Psychiatric/Mental Health
A ADHD in Children and Adults ....8 hrs
Antidepressants ....1 hr
Antipsychotics ....1 hr
Anxiolytics and Mood Stabilizers ....1 hr
Basic Psychopharmacology ....5 hrs
Behavioral Approaches to Treating Obesity.....................13 hrs
A Bipolar Disorder ....10 hrs
A Borderline Personality Disorder ....21 hrs
A Child/Adolescent Clinical Psychopharmacology ....12 hrs
A Childhood Maltreatment..10 hrs
A Clinical Psychopharmacology ....10 hrs
A Collaborative Therapy with Multi-stressed Families ....30 hrs
Depression: Prevention, Diagnosis, and Treatment ....25 hrs
A Evidence-Based Mental Health Practice............................22 hrs
A Geropsychiatric and Mental Health Nursing ....40 hrs
A Integrating Traditional Healing Practices ....35 hrs
IPV (Intimate Partner Violence) (2nd ed.) ....1 or 3 hrs
A Mental Disorders in Older Adults.....................................25 hrs
A Mindfulness and Psychotherapy.......................................25 hrs
A Multicultural Perspectives in Working with Families ....27 hrs
A Obsessive Compulsive Disorder..9 hrs
A Problem and Pathological Gambling ....9 hrs
Psychiatric Nursing: Current Trends in Diagnosis ....30 hrs
Psychiatric Principles & Applications ....30 hrs
A Schizophrenia ....5 hrs
Substance Abuse ....32 hrs
A Suicide..21 hrs
A Trauma Therapy ....11 hrs
A Treating Explosive Kids ....14 hrs
A Treating Victims of Mass Disaster and Terrorism ....6 hrs

REV. 1/20/08